SPEECH AND LANGUAGE DISORDERS

DYSLEXIA

ANALYSIS AND
CLINICAL SIGNIFICANCE

SPEECH AND LANGUAGE DISORDERS

Additional books and e-books in this series can be found on Nova's website under the Series tab.

SPEECH AND LANGUAGE DISORDERS

DYSLEXIA

ANALYSIS AND CLINICAL SIGNIFICANCE

CATIA GIACONI

AND

SIMONE APARECIDA CAPELLINI

EDITORS

nova
Medicine & Health
New York

Copyright © 2020 by Nova Science Publishers, Inc.

All rights reserved. No part of this book may be reproduced, stored in a retrieval system or transmitted in any form or by any means: electronic, electrostatic, magnetic, tape, mechanical photocopying, recording or otherwise without the written permission of the Publisher.

We have partnered with Copyright Clearance Center to make it easy for you to obtain permissions to reuse content from this publication. Simply navigate to this publication's page on Nova's website and locate the "Get Permission" button below the title description. This button is linked directly to the title's permission page on copyright.com. Alternatively, you can visit copyright.com and search by title, ISBN, or ISSN.

For further questions about using the service on copyright.com, please contact:
Copyright Clearance Center
Phone: +1-(978) 750-8400   Fax: +1-(978) 750-4470   E-mail: info@copyright.com

NOTICE TO THE READER

The Publisher has taken reasonable care in the preparation of this book, but makes no expressed or implied warranty of any kind and assumes no responsibility for any errors or omissions. No liability is assumed for incidental or consequential damages in connection with or arising out of information contained in this book. The Publisher shall not be liable for any special, consequential, or exemplary damages resulting, in whole or in part, from the readers' use of, or reliance upon, this material. Any parts of this book based on government reports are so indicated and copyright is claimed for those parts to the extent applicable to compilations of such works.

Independent verification should be sought for any data, advice or recommendations contained in this book. In addition, no responsibility is assumed by the Publisher for any injury and/or damage to persons or property arising from any methods, products, instructions, ideas or otherwise contained in this publication.

This publication is designed to provide accurate and authoritative information with regard to the subject matter covered herein. It is sold with the clear understanding that the Publisher is not engaged in rendering legal or any other professional services. If legal or any other expert assistance is required, the services of a competent person should be sought. FROM A DECLARATION OF PARTICIPANTS JOINTLY ADOPTED BY A COMMITTEE OF THE AMERICAN BAR ASSOCIATION AND A COMMITTEE OF PUBLISHERS.

Additional color graphics may be available in the e-book version of this book.

Library of Congress Cataloging-in-Publication Data

ISBN: 978-1-53617-593-6

Published by Nova Science Publishers, Inc. † New York

CONTENTS

Preface		ix
Chapter 1	Use of Assistive Technology in Reading Intervention with Dyslexia *Maíra Anelli Martins,* *Adriana Marques de Oliveira* *and Simone Aparecida Capellini*	1
Chapter 2	Clinical Significance Analysis of Metaphonological Performance and Reading in School Children with Mixed Dyslexia after Intervention: Case Study *Gabriela Franco dos Santos Liporaci* *and Simone Aparecida Capellini*	15
Chapter 3	Tier 2 Response to Intervention (RTI) Model: Intervention with Alphabetical Principle and Metaphonological Skills *Alexandra Beatriz Portes de Cerqueira César,* *Melissa Pinotti Marguti* *and Simone Aparecida Capellini*	29

Chapter 4	Analysis of the Clinical Significance of Students with Dyslexia in Reading Process Evaluation *Isabela Pires Metzner and Simone Aparecida Capellini*	**43**
Chapter 5	Clinical Significance of Text Reading Comprehension after Remediation with Rapid Naming and Reading *Bianca dos Santos and Simone Aparecida Capellini*	**59**
Chapter 6	Dyslexia and Chinese Language: A Case Study *Catia Giaconi, Simone Aparecida Capellini, Noemi Del Bianco and Ilaria D'Angelo*	**71**
Chapter 7	Clinical Significance of Perceptual-Motor Performance and Handwriting of Students with Mixed Subtype Dyslexia *Larissa Sellin, Isabela Pires Metzner and Simone Aparecida Capellini*	**83**
Chapter 8	Characterization of Fine Motor Function in Students with Developmental Dyslexia *Giseli Donadon Germano, Raíssa Angleni Machado Pereira and Simone Aparecida Capellini*	**95**
Chapter 9	Visual Perception Studies in the Italian Language *Ilaria DÁngelo, Noemi Del Bianco, Simone Aparecida Capellini and Catia Giaconi*	**109**

Chapter 10	Dyslexia in the University System: Technology for Autonomy *Noemi Del Bianco, Catia Giaconi,* *Ilaria D'Angelo* *and Simone Aparecida Capellini*	**119**
Editors' Contact Information		**133**
Index		**135**

PREFACE

Dyslexia: Analysis and Clinical Significance is a book composed by ten chapters with scientific contributions in the fields of Speech Language Pathology and Education about case study on Dyslexia.

Martins, Oliveira and Capellini present the first chapter on "Use of Assistive Technology in Reading Intervention with Dyslexia." The second chapter is from Liporaci and Capellini on "Clinical Significance Analysis of Metaphonological Performance and Reading in School Children with Mixed Dyslexia after Intervention: Case Study." César, Marguti and Capellini wrote the third chapter on "Tier 2 Response to Intervention (RTI) Model: Intervention with Alphabetical Principle and Metaphonological Skills."

The fourth chapter is from Metzner and Capellini on "Analysis of the Clinical Significance of Students with Dyslexia in Reading Process Evaluation." Santos and Capellini present the fifth contribution on "Clinical Significance of Text Reading Comprehension after Remediation with Rapid Naming and Reading." The sixth contribution is written by Giaconi, Capellini and Del Bianco entitled "Dyslexia and Chinese Language: A Case Study."

Sellin, Metzner and Capellini present the seventh contribution on "Clinical Significance of Perceptual-Motor Performance and Handwriting of Students with Mixed Subtype Dyslexia." The contribution

"Characterization of Fine Motor Function in Students with Developmental Dyslexia" is the eighth chapter by Germano, Pereira and Capellini. The ninth chapter on "Visual Perception studies in Italian Language" is from D'Angelo, Del Bianco, Capellini and Giaconi.

The tenth and final contribution entitled "Dyslexia in University System: Technology for Autonomy" is from Del Bianco, Giaconi and Capellini.

We conclude this preface wishing a good reading for everyone!!

Catia Giaconi
Simone Aparecida Capellini
Editors

In: Dyslexia　　　　　　　　　　　ISBN: 978-1-53617-593-6
Editors: Catia Giaconi et al.　　© 2020 Nova Science Publishers, Inc.

Chapter 1

USE OF ASSISTIVE TECHNOLOGY IN READING INTERVENTION WITH DYSLEXIA

Maíra Anelli Martins, Adriana Marques de Oliveira and Simone Aparecida Capellini

Investigation Learning Disabilities Laboratory (LIDA),
Department of Speech and Hearing Sciences,
São Paulo State University "Júlio de Mesquita Filho" (UNESP),
Marilia, São Paulo, Brazil

INTRODUCTION

According to the most important diagnostic manual used for the assessment criteria - *Diagnostic and Statistical Manual of Mental Disorders (DSM-V)* dyslexia is a specific neurodevelopmental disorder and its major manifestations regarding learning disabilities firstly shows during the school years. In some cases, however, they manifest when academic demands exceed the limited capabilities of the scholar. Thus, their manifestations are more visible during the literacy process, affecting the teaching and learning process, and may also affect the entire professional and emotional trajectory during school life (American Psychiatry Association - APA, 2013).

Dyslexia is a multifaceted disorder, which may explain why a single universally accepted definition has not yet been reached. This fact makes the diagnosis of this disorder more challenging, considering that dyslexia manifests heterogeneously in both behavioral and cognitive criteria (Lyon, Shaywitz & Shaywitz, 2003).

Learning disabilities are persistent and non-transient, despite intense and appropriate remediation instruction given to children and adolescents, yet difficulties with fluent accuracy and/or word recognition, poor spelling and decoding skills persist, preventing the individual from achieving the same level of reading ability as other students in their class group. Secondary consequences may also include problems with reading comprehension and reduced reading experience, affecting the development of vocabulary and prior knowledge (Moojen, Bassôa, & Gonçalves, 2016).

Dyslexia impacts the psychosocial life of individuals and may be associated with anxiety and depression resulting from social, emotional and behavioral problems. Low self-esteem and lack of motivation are also observed in students with dyslexia (Hendren, Haft, Black, White, & Hoeft, 2018).

Since motivation is one of the important aspects of the learning process, creating and reinventing strategies that motivate these students and enable them to engage in reading and writing activities is a challenge, especially when students want to be authors of their own learning process, besides overcoming their difficulties. This reinvention seeks to combine game and technology schemes to help in this process.

The technological evolution once assimilated into our routine to favor daily activities is understood today as an aid to promote the expansion of a deficient functional ability, or to allow the desired accomplishment, which is hindered by the circumstance of deficiency or aging, called assistive technology (Radabaugh, 1993). Assistive technology is the use of resources and services to alleviate functional problems faced by individuals with disabilities, and to provide or expand their skills, thus promoting greater independence, quality of life, social inclusion, learning ability, work, and inclusion (integration with family, friends and society) (Technical Assistance Committee, 2007; Sameshima & Silva, 2012).

The American with Disabilities (ACT) (ADA, 1994) defines assistive technology resources as any and all items, equipment or parts, products or systems manufactured in series or tailored to increase, maintain, or enhance the functional capabilities of people with disabilities. The use of technology enables the more efficient teaching of reading and writing skills and promotes the involvement and interest of students with dyslexia in reading and writing activities (Berninger et al., 2015; Bjekic et al., 2014; Cidrin & Madeiro, 2017; Defior., & Serrano, 2011; Lysenko & Abrami, 2014; Mousinho, 2009; Skiada et al., 2014; Zapata, Zikl, et al., 2015).

Reid (2013) states that students with dyslexia learn more efficiently when material is presented visually and have the opportunity to kinesthetically interact with it. Therefore, it must be ensured that teaching and learning are multisensory since it is a key aspect of successful learning for dyslexic scholars. The author explains that multisensory learning involves hearing, vision, kinesthesia, and tactile input, and that it can be offered by computers and tablets. Thus, in order to facilitate the orientation to the use of technological resources, it is suggested the division by skills for better visualization of resources, tools, and strategies, such as Reading, Metacognitive Skills, Writing, Notes and Study, and Organizational Skills.

READING

The major and most important difference of technology in the therapeutic and teaching process is the individualization in resource use planning, as stated by Foz and Picarone (2014). According to the authors, these activities can be performed with a computer and software such as Microsoft Office PowerPoint. The authors, for instance, present strategies that work on developing reading fluency (speed, accuracy, and prosody) using this type of feature.

Proven strategies to foster the development of reading and writing can be incorporated into the use of tools such as tablets and laptops, and repeated reading strategy, which can be applied along with recorder-aided reading modeling (Hotchcock, Prater, & Dowrick, 2004).

Using audiobooks can also be a worthy tool to support corrective feedback, modeling, and repeated timed reading strategies. The student can study models of fluent readings by listening to audiobooks, later record their oral reading, and then listen to their recording and perform their corrections and self-monitoring by counting correct and incorrect words per minute. This activity allows for an efficient practice experience to improve fluency with minimal use of human advice. For students who need more support, video-assisted reading can be done. Here students read aloud simultaneously or as an echo with an audio-recorded model (Hotchcock, Prater, & Dowrick, 2004). The authors proved in their study that video self-modeling speeds up reading fluency skills and strengthens reading comprehension.

Computers can be effectively used to provide reading fluency practices. There are efforts by researchers to develop web pages and software that offer appropriate reading material in which strategies with metalinguistic skills, spelling, vocabulary, fluency, and reading comprehension can be worked on, including game-like activities with feedback. Besides, computers can assist with applications that scan adult dyslexic reading. There are mobile and tablet apps, for instance, that offer thousands of audiobooks, e-books, podcasts, magazines, and newspapers, as well as software and applications that read written materials. It is also possible to find software that converts scanned material into a text file to be read aloud by the computer.

In addition to reading the text (you can determine the reading speed), you can also highlight each section in a different color while reading it, and highlight each word you want while the process is in progress. When students can hear unfamiliar words read (without asking the teacher or a colleague), reading speed and comprehension can dramatically improve. Also, using speech synthesis technology in elementary and high school classrooms can help students with low self-esteem, and by decoding difficulties they become more independent readers, helping them to experience successful reading and better comprehension. (Forgrave, 2002). There are also features to increase the font size, change the font, increase spacing and move the text in different directions, as well as dictionary functions (Shaywitz, 2006).

WRITING

There is also software that reads texts in PDF, Docx, TXT and ePub extensions for the listener. Many also allow you to change the reading speed and the reader's voice. There are a variety of computer products that can help with voice recognition, spell checking and voice feedback, and even write dictated text. To work with writing, speech recognition programs can be complemented by other software that reads aloud and pronounces typed words, verifying that the person has typed the intended word. Programs were developed to convert spoken text into written text, that is, to convert oral language into digital format. These tools offer ways for students to engage with writing, assisting them with text production, as well as assisting with grammar and spelling review (Foz & Picarone, 2014; Reid, 2013). Prediction activities (complete the gaps) of a letter in words, or syllables in words and words in sentences can be performed by software. It is also possible to work on syllable manipulations, spelling training and handwriting activities using appropriate gadgets.

Admittedly, there are different devices and applications for students with all kinds of special needs, however, this is not yet a reality for many countries. Researchers argue about the popularity of mobile technology which includes smartphones, mp3 players such as the iPod and tablet computers. Nevertheless, in countries such as Brazil, for example, mobile technologies are restricted to mobile phones, which most of the population can access, including children. On the other hand, the good news is that there is a growth in the development of applications that can be downloaded and used for free on these more affordable mobile devices. Apps make it possible to individualize teaching, learning, and communication (Reid, Strnadová, & Cumming, 2013). The ability to customize a popular device to suit each student's needs is motivating because it gives them something dominant and stigma-free, yet engaging and interactive.

METACOGNITIVE SKILLS

Regarding the skills of syllabic analysis, it is possible to work with phonological awareness in oral language by using a tape recorder and a game scheme. It is necessary to draw up decks of letters with the letters of the alphabet, and record the sounds of the syllables, as well as a record sheet for the words and phrases that the student forms. The student is asked to select ten letters and form a word using the letters he drew. Then you have to split the word into syllables and record (the syllable sound) on the recorder, each syllable will be recorded in a separate audio. For example, if the word has four syllables, there will be four different audios, one for each syllable. Subsequently, you list the audios to hear the recorded word of each audio. Finally, the student is asked to hear the syllables and repeat the word aloud, and then you register it on the answer sheet. When you are finished, write three sentences with the word formed, one declarative, one interrogative and one exclamatory phrase. In this activity, it is noted that the recorder, which is usually a cell phone, can be a multipurpose strategy, with several ways to use it (Silva, 2017).

At the beginning of literacy, guiding children to search for new words, especially those that find it difficult to read, is a strategy. Saying the word out loud helps you reach your phonological form, a pathway to its meaning, and for that, assistive technologies can be helpful. This is the case with computerized pens, where you can scan words in the text, and the word definition is shown on the pen display, and you can read it aloud.

You can also create strategies to teach the phonemes of the children's names at the PowerPoint: in shapes, select a box, write a grapheme, record the audio, and link to it. When you click the box, the sound is produced, which may be the phoneme or the letter name. You can also prepare rhyming activities and alliteration, among others.

NOTES AND STUDIES

Notes can be made using relatively inexpensive small keyboards with a small display that allows viewing many lines of written text. With the keyboard, you can take notes in class and save everything you write, and it can be connected to virtually any existing word processor. So when you get home, you can copy everything you wrote at school to your computer. With a palmtop, for instance, you can connect to a folding keyboard, which is useful for taking notes in class. Recording classes on a portable recorder or even on your cell phone is useful for storing information so you can access them whenever specific points need to be clarified, as well as recording your own work. You can make recordings of an essay that is intended to be written and later transcribe it with the help of a colleague, friend or teacher. With the help of speech recognition software, it is possible to record and listen to the rehearsal for later modification as the digital copy is produced (Shaywitz, 2005).

As a result of a phonological deficit, dyslexic readers experience difficulties with handwriting and spelling, and challenges in decoding words (converting graphemes into phonemes) rise when trying to do the opposite process: writing correctly, which depends on the coding of sounds and their transformation into letters. Spell checkers help a lot, as do the software that specializes in this work (Shaywitz, 2005). Using visual organizers (for example, online semantic maps) to plan the writing process improves the quality of writing by helping students summarize the information they read. Organizational programs also facilitate the understanding process by creating a visual format that reflects the relationships between text ideas or key concepts (Forgrave, 2002).

ORGANIZATIONAL SKILLS

Being organized is a skill that many students may experience difficulties, and those with dyslexia may have even more. Time organization, task planning, and general work can be challenging for students with dyslexia. Some applications allow students to track time and plan activities efficiently.

However, we highlight here a 15-year review study on the use of assistive technology by MacArthur, Ferretti, Okolo & Cavalier (2001) in which it has been shown that only use or exposure to assistive technology is not sufficient to improve dramatically improve students' literacy skills and competences. Some students, especially those with dyslexia or reading and writing learning disorders, require explicit and systematic teaching of these skills that may be associated with the use of technology. Professionals must be able to integrate assistive technology to maximize student success.

FINAL CONSIDERATIONS

With the increasing amount of digitally distributed information and the innovation of technology, there are more and more resources to build programs for working with students with dyslexia, whether individualized or collective, for clinical, group or classroom work. The use of assistive technology enables dyslexic students to read information, organize their ideas and write more clearly. Thus, with the use of technology, students have the means to complete well-written and organized tasks that can truly reflect their knowledge and skills.

With these innovations, it is possible to motivate and lead the student to greater engagement in reading and writing activities. However, it is emphasized that it is necessary to look at the difficulties that the student presents so that teachers, professionals, and parents can search among several technological resources that are appropriate for each school.

REFERENCES

Acheampong, P., & Acquaah, P. A. (2015). Talking books technique: a strategy to improve pupils' reading and comprehension skills. *European Journal of Research and Reflection in Educational Sciences, 3*(2), 1-17.

ADA - American with Disabilities ACT 1994. Disponível em: http://www.resna.org/taproject/library/laws/techact94.htm Acesso em 05/10/2007.

American Psychiatric Association (2013). *Diagnostic and Statistical Manual of Mental Disorders, Fifth Edition* – DSM -5. Arlington, VA: American Psychiatric Association Publishing.

Berninger, V. W., Nagy, W., Tanimoto, S., & Thompson R. D., Abbott, R. (2015). Computer instruction in handwriting, spelling, and composing for students with specific learning disabilities in grades 4-9. *Computers & Education*, 81, 154-168. doi:10.1016/j.compedu.2014.10.005.

Bjekic, D., Obradovic, S., Vucetic, M., & Bojovic, M. (2014). E-teacher in inclusive e-education for students with specific learning desabilities. *Procedia - Social and Behavioral Sciences*, *128*(22), 128-133. https://doi.org/10.1016/j.sbspro.2014.03.131.

CAT - Comitê de Ajudas Técnicas. *Ata da Reunião III, de abril de 2007 do Comitê de Ajudas Técnicas.* Secretaria Especial dos Direitos Humanos da Presidência da República (CORDE/SEDH/PR), 2007. Disponível em: < http://www.mj.gov.br/corde/comite.asp. Acesso em: 29 out. 2019. [Technical Assistance Committe. Minutes of Meeting III, April 2007, of the Technical Assistance Committee. Special Secretary for Human Rights of the Presidency of the Republic (CORDE/SEDH/PR), 2007. Retrieved from: < http://www.mj.gov.br/corde/comite.asp. cited: 2019 oct 2009.]

Forgrave, K. E. (2002). Assistive technology: empowering students with learning disabilities. *The Clearing House*, 75(3), 122-126, doi: 10.1080/00098650209599250.

Foz, F. B., & Picarone, M. L. C. D. (2014). Uso de tecnologias na intervenção nos problemas de aprendizagem. IN: M. A. Martins. M. H. Cardoso, & S. A. Capellini. *Tópicos em Transtornos de aprendizagem parte III.* (pp. 153-171). Marília: Fundepe: Cultura Acadêmica. [Use of technologies to intervention in learning disabilities. IN: M. A. Martins. M. H. Cardoso, & S. A. Capellini.

Topics in Learning Disabilities part III. ((pp. 153-171). Marília: Fundepe: Academic Culture].

Hendren, R. L., Haft, S. L., Black, J. M., White, N. C., & Hoeft, F. (2018). Recognizing Psychiatric Comorbidity with Reading Disorders. *Frontiers in psychiatry, 9*(101), 1-10. doi: 10.3389/fpsyt. 2018.00101. eCollection 2018.

Hitchocock, C. H., Prater, M. A., & Dowricl, P. W. (2004). Reading comprehension and fluency: examining the effects of tutoring and video self-modeling on first-grade students with reading difficulties. *Learning Disability Quaterly, 27,* 89-103. https://doi.org/10. 2307/1593644.

Koulopoulou, A. (2010). P01-221 - Anxiety and depression symptoms in children-commorbidity with learning disabilities. *European Psychiatry, 25*(1), 432. https://doi.org/10.1016/S0924-9338(10) 70427-2.

Lock, R. H., & Welsch, R. G. (2006). Increase Oral Reading Fluency. *Intervention in School and Clinic, 41*(3), *180*-183. doi.org/10.1177/ 10534512060410030901.

Lopes, A. M. (2017). Aprendendo com as letras. In: *Tecnologias com sentido.* A. Pinheiro & R. Ramalho (Ogs). Editora Paula Frassinetti.

Lyon, G. R., Shaywitz, S. E., & Shaywitz, B. A. (2003). A definition of dyslexia. *Annals of Dyslexia. 53*(1), 1-14.

Lysenko, L. V., & Abrami, P. C. (2014). Promoting reading comprehension with the use of technology. *Computers & Education*, 75, 162-172. https://doi.org/10.1016/j.compedu.2014.01. 010.

MacArthur, C. A., R. P. Ferretti, C. M. Okolo, & A. R. Cavalier. (2001). Technology applications for students with literacy problems: a critical review. *The Elementary School Journal 101*(3), 273-301. Retrieved from http://www.jstor.org/stable/1002248.

Moojen, S. M. P, Bassôa, A., & Gonçalves, H. A. (2016). *Characteristics of development dyslexia and its manifestation in adulthood.* Psychopedagogy Journal, *33*(100), 50-59.

Mousinho, R. Dislexia e inclusão: possibilidades de adaptações metodológicas e adaptativas. In: A. Lamoglia. (Eds). *Temas em inclusão. Saberes e práticas.* (pp. 1-15.) Rio de Janeiro: Unirio Synergia; 2009. [Dyslexia and inclusion: possibilities of adaptations methodological and adaptive. In: A. Lamoglia. (Eds). *Inclusion themes: Knowledge and practices.* (pp. 1-15.) Rio de Janeiro: Unirio Synergia; 2009].

Radabaugh, M. P. (1993). *NIDRR's Long Range Plan* - Technology for Access and Function Research Section Two: NIDDR.

Reid, G., Strnadová, I., & Cumming, T. (2013). Expanding horizons for students with dyslexia in the 21st century: universal design and mobile technology. *Journal of Research in Special Educational Needs, 13*(3), 175-181.

Research Agenda Chapter 5: Technology for Access and Function - http://www.ncddr.org/rpp/techaf/lrp_ov.html.

Sameshima, F. A., & Silva, F. R. P. (2012). Implementation of assistive techology resources and procedures in specialized educational services. *Scientific Journal of Unisalesiano – Academical, 3*(6), 69-78.

Shaywitz, S. (2005). *Overcoming Dyslexia: A New complete science-based program for reading problems at any level.* New York: Vintage Books.

Silva, R. (2017). Qual a letra que ganha? In: A. Pinheiro & R. Ramalho (Eds). *Tecnologias com sentido.* Editora Paula Frassinetti. [Which letter wins? In: A. Pinheiro & R. Ramalho (Eds). Tecnologies with meaning. Publisher Paula Frassinetti].

Skiada, R., Soroniati, E., Gardeli, A., & Zissis, D. (2014). EasyLexia: a mobile application for children with learning difficulties. *Procedia Computer Science, 27,* 218-228. https://doi.org/10.1016/j.procs.2014.02.025.

Zapata, E. G., Defior, S., & Serrano, F. (2011). Improving reading fluency in dyslexia: designing a Spanish intervention program. *Writtings of Psychology, 4*(2), 65-73. Cited: 2019 Nov 04.

Retrieved from: http://scielo.isciii.es/scielo.php?script=sci_arttext&pid=S1989-38092011000200008&lng=es&tlng=es.

Zikl, P. et al., (2015). The possibilities of ICT use for compensation of difficulties with reading in pupils with dyslexia. *Procedia - Social and Behavioral Sciences, 176,* 915-922. https://doi.org/10.1016/j.sbspro.2015.01.558.

In: Dyslexia
Editors: Catia Giaconi et al.

ISBN: 978-1-53617-593-6
© 2020 Nova Science Publishers, Inc.

Chapter 2

CLINICAL SIGNIFICANCE ANALYSIS OF METAPHONOLOGICAL PERFORMANCE AND READING IN SCHOOL CHILDREN WITH MIXED DYSLEXIA AFTER INTERVENTION: CASE STUDY

Gabriela Franco dos Santos Liporaci
and Simone Aparecida Capellini
Investigation Learning Disabilities Laboratory (LIDA),
Department of Speech and Hearing Sciences,
São Paulo State University "Júlio de Mesquita Filho" (UNESP),
Marilia, São Paulo, Brazil

INTRODUCTION

Dyslexia refers to differences in individual processing, often characterized by the difficulties presented at the beginning of literacy, compromising the acquisition of reading, writing and spelling. Cognitive, phonological and/or visual processes may also fail (Reid 2016). Thus, it is a specific learning disorder of neurological origin, characterized by difficulty with correct reading fluency and difficulty in decoding and spelling ability, resulting from a deficit in the phonological component of language (Lyon; Shaywitz; Shaywitz 2003).

Reading is one of the most important inputs to knowledge, as it is necessary for learning the content proposed by both academia and daily life situations. This implies the importance of acquiring reading ability, which is considered a multisensory difficulty, in which the reader has to combine a visual element (grapheme) with an auditory element (phoneme) in a new audiovisual unit. Simultaneously, the reader must also learn to extract a specific phoneme from the auditory input, in another continuous way, to create a new representation of the phoneme which also includes its orthographic characteristic (Schlesinger; Gray 2017), for reading is conceived as the main tool for the students to acquire new concepts and one of the biggest challenges of the school in the present times (Bandini et al. 2014; Cain et al. 2001; Fonseca-Mora 2015; Morais 2013; Navas; Pinto; Delissa 2009; Norton et al. 2014; Oakhill; Cain 2012; Oliveira; Capellini 2016).

Alphabetical principle is the principle of representation of language phonemes by letters or graphemes, that is, the knowledge that graphic forms represent phonemic segments of speech, in which a given phoneme can be represented by a specific letter. The alphabet is a writing system in which individual or group characters represent phonemes, even if the spelling code introduces considerable variability in the grapheme-phoneme relationship (Morais 2013; Snowling; Hulme 2013). It is important to bear in mind that the basis of the Portuguese writing system is the letter and not the syllables as stated by Cagliari (1996, p. 119) "although our writing contains numbers, acronyms, ideographic signs, etc., it is fundamentally based on the letter".

It is important to be clear about what letter, sound, grapheme and phoneme are, as these terms are often used as synonyms when they are not. The letter is defined as the graphic representation of the signs or graphic signs present in the alphabet (set of letters) that represent the phonemes of speech.

There are 26 letters to represent the written Portuguese language. Sound, in turn, is nothing more than the acoustic energy that results from periodic and non-periodic vibrations of the phonatory apparatus structures. Provided the sound in assigned the function of 38 distinct functions, it is called phoneme. The phoneme is the smallest phonological unit that distinguishes meaning.

Therefore, they are abstract, elementary, and distinctive sounds that correspond to each letter, while the grapheme consists of one or more letters representing a phoneme, and also has the function of distinguishing meanings. In the alphabetical system of Brazilian Portuguese, there are 72 number of graphemes, and they have no more than two letters, with or without graphic accents (Cagliari 1996; Cegalla 2008; Cuetos 2010; Dehaene 2012; Gabriel; Morais; Kolinsky 2016; Morais 2013; Scliar-Cabral 2003; 2008; 2013b; Snowling; Hulme 2013; Soares 2003).

Students with better mastery of metaphonological skills begin to learn to read more easily than other students, whereas students who have deficiencies in these skills tend to have significant reading difficulties (Farris et al. 2016; Saksida et al. 2016).

Thus, metaphonological skills are necessary for reading and writing, as phonological awareness will be an aspect to be integrated into word recognition.

Written language should be considered as a system of language representation, whose learning means the appropriation of a new object of knowledge. It is necessary to understand that the structure of the alphabetic system of Portuguese does not mean that the writing of this system is the graphic representation of its sounds, but that the perception of sounds during the production of oral language directly influences development of reading and writing (Capellini and Oliveira 2003).

Metaphonological skills concern the identification and production of rhyme and alliteration, word segmentation (lexical segmentation), syllable word segmentation and phoneme word segmentation (phonemic segmentation). These skills differ in the level of cognitive demand (Stanovich 1992).

Research that incorporates intervention programs into metaphonological skills demonstrates the influences of this skill on the process of written language acquisition (Ball and blachman 1991; Bradley and bryant 1983; Lundberg, Frost and petersen 1988; Torgesen and Davis 1996; Torgesen, Morgan and Davis 1992; Torgesen, Wagner, Rashotte et al. 1999; Santos 2010).

Thus, metaphonological skills are necessary for reading and writing, as phonological awareness will be an aspect to be integrated into word recognition (Capellini and Oliveira 2003).

Thus, we must consider that intervention programs for students with developmental dyslexia should contain the specificities of each subtype of dyslexia. The mixed subtype of developmental dyslexia is one that presents alterations in auditory, visual and sequential processing, causing difficulties in the use of reading routes.

This chapter aims to present the analysis of the clinical significance of the performance of students with mixed dyslexia in metaphonological and reading skills, based on scientific evidence.

METHOD

The study included three students diagnosed with mixed dyslexia who underwent pre-testing and post-testing (Table 1).

Next, we will present the Metalinguistic and Reading Skills Protocol (Cunha; Capellini 2009) that was used to verify the analysis of the clinical significance of the subjects after intervention, in a post-test situation.

Table 1. Distribution of students submitted to pre-intervention and post-test pilot study according to gender, age and grade

Identification	Group	Diagnostic	Series
S1	Pilot	Dylexia	5th Year
S2	Pilot	Dyslexia	4th Year
S3	Pilot	Dyslexia	4th Year

Protocol Metalinguistic Skills Testing and Reading - PROHMELE (Cunha, Capellini 2009)

Composed by the following tests:

- *Syllabic and phonemic identification tests:* Initial syllable identification (ISI), Initial phoneme identification (IFI), Final syllable identification (ISF), Final phoneme identification (IFF), Medial syllable identification (ISM), medial phoneme (MFI).
- *Tests of syllabic and phonemic manipulation:* Segmentation (SegSil), Segmentation (SegFon), Addition (Ad Sil), Addition (Ad Fon), Substitution (SubsSil), Substitution (SubsFon), Subtraction (SubtFon), Syllable Combination (With Sil), Phoneme Combination (With Fon).
- *Reading Tests:* Reading of real words: list of isolated real words (133 words); Reading pseudo words: list of pseudo words (27 pseudo words)

The application of the tests of metalinguistic skills was performed so that the student did not get visual clue of the articulation of sounds produced by the evaluator. The characterization of the types of errors of reading real words and pseudo words were performed from the raw score of each test.

Table 2. Performance of subjects in the PROHMELE Metalinguistic and Reading Skills Test Protocol tests

Subjects	ISI	IFI	ISF	IFF	ISM	IFM	SUB S	SUB F	AS	AF	SBS S	SBS F	CS	CF	SS	SF
1	-	-	-	-	-	-	-	-	-	-	-	-	-	-	-	-
2	-	-	-	-	-	-	-	-	-	-	-	-	-	-	-	-
3	-	-	-	-	-	-	-	-	MPC	-	MPC	-	-	-	-	-

Caption: ISI = initial syllable identification; IFI = initial phoneme identification; ISF = final syllable identification; IFF = final phoneme identification; ISM = medial syllable identification; MFI = medial phoneme identification; SUB S = syllable replacement; SUB F = phoneme substitution; AS = syllable addition; AF = phoneme addition; SBS S = syllable subtraction; SBS F = phoneme subtraction; CS = syllable combination; CF = phoneme combination; SS = syllable segmentation; SF = phoneme segmentation; MPC = reliable positive change; MNC = reliable negative change.

RESULTS

The individual analysis was performed using the JT Method, which performs the comparative analysis between pre and post intervention scores, in order to decide two complementary processes, which are the reliable change index and the clinical significance of the changes (Jacobson; Truax 1991; Del Prette; Del Prette 2008, Apud Santos 2017). Thus, the results of this study will be presented below.

In Table 2, we can see that subject 3 presented reliable positive change (MPC) in addition of syllables and presented positive positive change (MPC) in the syllable replacement test.

In table 3 it was possible to observe reliable positive change (MPC) in subjects 1, 2 and 3, which presented respectively positive positive change (MPC) in the word reading and pseudoword reading tests.

In Table 4 it was possible to observe reliable positive change (MPC) in subjects 2 and 3. Subject 2 presented MPC in repetition of non-monosyllabic words.

Subject 3 presented MPC in repetition of non-three-syllable words, with four and five syllables.

Table 3. Performance of EG subjects in the word and pseudoword tests of the Metalinguistic and Reading Skills Test Protocol – PROHMELE

	1	MPC
LP	2	MPC
	3	MPC
	1	MPC
LPP	2	MPC
	3	MPC

Caption: LP = word reading;
LPP = pseudoword reading;
MPC = reliable positive change;
MNC = reliable negative change.

Table 4. Performance of GE subjects in the non-word repetition tests of the PROHMELE Reading and Metalinguistic Testing Protocol

Subject	RNP_M	RNP_D	RNP_T	RNP_P4	RNP_P5	RNP_P6
1	-	-	-	-	-	-
2	MPC	-	-	-	-	-
3	-	-	MPC	MPC	MPC	MPC

Caption: RNP_M = repetition of non-monosyllabic words; RNP_D = repetition of non-syllable words; RNP_T = repetition of non-trisyllabic words; RNP_4 = non-word repetition with four syllables; RNP_5 = non-word repetition with five syllables; RNP_6 = non-word repetition with six syllables.

In summary, based on these data it is possible to conclude that, regarding the Metalinguistic Skills Protocol - PROHMELE (Cunha; Capellini 2009), the individual S1 of the pilot group, submitted to the Phonological Intervention Program associated with reading and writing for students with dyslexia, presented positive change in the reading time of real words and showed no change in the non-word repetition test.

The subject S2, on the other hand, presented reliable positive change in word and pseudo word reading and repetition of non-monosyllabic words.

Subject S3 showed reliable positive change in syllable addition and syllable substitution, real and pseudo word reading and non-trisyllabic word repetition, four-syllable non-polysyllabic word repetition, five-syllable non-polysyllabic word repetition.

DISCUSSION

The importance of teaching metaphonological skills in both educational and clinical contexts is evident in children who learn based on the alphabetic principle, since there is a study (Barrera and Santos 2014) that shows that metaphonological skills favor and facilitate reading and writing skills and that these skills can be developed through intervention programs.

When referring to metaphonological skills, it cannot be ruled out that in addition to difficulties in developing written language, difficulties related to oral language also occur (Preston and Edwards 2010). Assuming that the assessment of these skills includes reflecting on the sounds and manipulating them, when a child shows difficulty it means that the child has difficulty in understanding small units of language (Frost et al. 2009).

Through this direct relationship with speech, it is possible to observe the development of these metaphonological skills even before the child enters school, but other skills, especially phonemic skills, will be acquired along with the literacy process of the student and consequently will learn the rules of the alphabetic system in Portuguese writing (Germano and Capellini 2015; Oliveira, Germano and Capellini 2017).

Observing the results of this study, it corroborates the reciprocal relationship between reading and writing learning and writing acquisition and different levels and skills in phonological awareness. Repetition tasks of non-words require skills to perceive, maintain and reproduce phonological information. Consequently, our findings indicate that the children responded positively after intervention, in which the students did not need a new exposure so that these skills could be performed. Previous research has shown that there is a relationship between working memory and performance in phonological awareness tasks (Alloway; Gathercole and Adams 2004).

There was also a significant change in relation to the reading of words and pseudo words, which we can affirm that, for reading to be stablished, the student has to perform the decoding and comprehension. Decoding is described in the literature as a skill related to the recognition of graphic symbols, which are represented by letters and words, which involves the perceptual skills (understanding and interpretation of graphic symbols from visual stimuli), identifying letters and the lexicon (linguistic knowledge of words, from which readers construct their meanings) (Cueto, 2010; Cunha; Oliveira 2010; Fonseca-Mora 2015; Giangiacomo; Navas 2008; Oliveira; Martins; Cunha 2015; Sánchez; García; Gonzales 2007).

Comprehension is the process by which words, sentences or texts are interpreted. It involves syntactic processes (knowledge of grammatical structures, which allows us to understand how words relate) and semantic processes (integration of current information - words, phrases or texts - with prior knowledge). Much of reading comprehension depends on one's prior knowledge (Cuetos 2010; Fonsecamora 2015; Giangiacomo; Navas 2008; Kintsch; Rawson 2013; Melgarejo et al. 2013; Morais 2013; Nation 2013; Perfetti; Landi; Oakhill 2013).

Decoding is the first step for automatic reading and is associated with reading comprehension performance, as fast and accurate word identification is essential and indispensable for reading comprehension. If the decoding step is automated, the readers can focus their efforts on the meaning of the material read. Thus, difficulties in comprehension may be the result of a general comprehension problem or an insufficient ability to identify written words (Bandini et al. 2014; Braze et al. 2016; Dehaene 2012; Kruk; Bergman 2013; Morais 2013; Nicolau, Navas 2015; Oliveira; Martins; Cunha 2015; Olson et al. 2013; Protopapas et al. 2013; Scliar-Cabral 2003).

Conclusion

The findings of this study revealed that the students showed improvement in syllabic manipulation activities and in the phonological decoding component of phonological working memory after the intervention, showing the development of the generative memory mechanism necessary for reading development.

REFERENCES

Cagliari, L.C. *Alfabetização & Linguística.* [*Literacy & Linguistics*] São Paulo (SP): Editora Scipione, 1996.

Cabral, L. S. (2003). *Princípios do sistema alfabético do português do Brasil.* [*Principles of the Brazilian Portuguese Alphabetical System*] Editora Contexto.

Capellini, A. S., & Oliveira, K. T. D. (2003). *Problemas de aprendizagem relacionados às alterações de linguagem. Distúrbios de aprendizagem: proposta de avaliação interdisciplinar.* [*Learning problems related to alterations in language. Learning disorders: proposal for an interdisciplinary assessment.*] São Paulo: Casa do Psicólogo, 113-139.

Cuetos, F., & Vega, F. C. (2010). *Psicología de la lectura.* [*Psychology of Reading*] WK Educación.

Cegalla, D. P. (1987). *Novíssima gramática da língua portuguesa:(con numerosos exercícios) para os alunos do 1 e 2 graus e para todos os estudiosos da língua nacional* [*New grammar of Portuguese language: (with numerous exercises) for 1st and 2nd grade students and for all students of the national language*]. Companhia Editora Nacional.

Cunha, V. L. O., & Capellini, S. A. (2009). Desempenho de escolares de 1ª a 4ª série do ensino fundamental nas provas de habilidades metafonológicas e de leitura-PROHMELE. [Performance of students from 1st to 4th grade of elementary school in the tests of metafonological and reading skills-PROHMELE] *Revista da Sociedade Brasileira de Fonoaudiologia*, 56-68.

Dehaene, S. (2012). *Os neurônios da leitura.* [*The neurons of Reading*] Porto Alegre: Penso.

Del Prette, Z. A. P., & Del Prette, A. (2008). Significância clínica e mudança confiável na avaliação de intervenções psicológicas. [Clinical significance and reliable change in the assessment of psychological interventions] *Psicologia: teoria e pesquisa,* 24(4), 497-505.

Fonseca-Mora, C. *Melodías en el proceso de desarrollo de la capacidad lectora.* [*Melodies inside the process of reading ability development.*] Revista de Estudios Filológicos, n. 25. Disponível em: Acesso em: 06 de jan. 2015.

Gabriel, R., Morais, J., & Kolinsky, R. (2016). A aprendizagem da leitura e suas implicações sobre a memória e a cognição. [The Learning process of reading and its implications to memory and cognition] *Ilha do Desterro: A Journal of English Language, Literatures in English and Cultural Studies,* 69(1), 61-78.

Germano, G. D., & Capellini, S. A. (2015). Avaliação das habilidades metafonológicas (PROHFON): caracterização e comparação do desempenho em escolares. [Evaluation of metaphonological skills (PROHFON): characterization and comparison of performance among scholars] *Psicologia: Reflexão e Crítica,* 28(2), 378-387. doi: 10.1590/1678-7153.201528218.

Hulme, C., & Showling, M. (2013). A ciência da leitura. [Science of Reading] *Porto Alegre: Penso,* 227-244.

Morais, J. (2013). *Criar leitores: para professores e educadores.* [*Raising readers: for teachers and educators*] São Paulo: Minha Editora.

Morais, J., Leite, I., & Kolinsky, R. (2013). Entre a pré-leitura e a leitura hábil: Condições e patamares da aprendizagem. [Between pre-reading and skillful reading: Apprenticeship conditions and levels] *Alfabetização no século XXI: Como se aprende a ler e a escrever* [*Literacy in the 21st century: How to learn to read and write*], 17-48.

Navas, A. L. G. P., Pinto, J. C. B. R., & Dellisa, P. R. R. (2009). *Avanços no conhecimento do processamento da fluência em leitura: da palavra ao texto.* [Advances in knowledge of fluency processing in reading: from word to text] Revista da Sociedade Brasileira de Fonoaudiologia.

Nicolau, C. C., & Navas, A. L. G. P. (2015). Avaliação das habilidades preditoras do sucesso de leitura em crianças de 1º e 2º anos do ensino fundamental. [Evaluation of the predictive skills of reading success in children from 1st and 2nd grades from elementary school. *Revista CEFAC*, 17(3), 917-926.

Oliveira, A. M. D., & Capellini, S. A. (2016, December). E-LEITURA II: banco de palavras para leitura de escolares do Ensino Fundamental II. [[E-Reading II: Word bank for middle schoolers reading] In *CoDAS* (Vol. 28, No. 6, pp. 778-817). Sociedade Brasileira de Fonoaudiologia.

Oliveira, A. M., Germano, G. D., & Capellini, S. A. (2017). Desempenho de escolares com dificuldades de aprendizagem em programa computadorizado de intervenção metafonológica e leitura. [Performance of students with learning difficulties with a computerized program of metaphonological intervention and Reading] *Psicologia Argumento*, 33(80).doi:10.7213/psicol.argum.33.080.AO01

Oliveira, A.M.; Martins, M.A.; Cunha, V.L.O. Relação entre decodificação, fluência, velocidade e compreensão de leitura. [Relationship between decoding, fluency, speed and reading comprehension] In: Andrade, O.V.C.A.; Okuda, P.M.M.; Capelini, S.A. (Ed) *Tópicos em Transtornos de aprendizagem parte IV* [*Topics in Learning Disorders part IV.*]. Marília (SP): Fundepe: Cultura Acadêmica, 2015. p. 41-53.

Santos, M. J., & Maluf, M. R. (2010). Consciência fonológica e linguagem escrita: efeitos de um programa de intervenção. [Phonological awareness and written language: effects of an intervention program] *Educar em revista*, (38), 57-71.

Soares, M. (2003). A reinvenção da alfabetização. [The reinvention of literacy] *Presença pedagógica*, 9(52), 15-21.

Scliar-Cabral, L. (2008). 2) Processamento bottom-up na leitura.[Bottom-up processing in Reading] Veredas-Revista de Estudos Linguísticos, 12(2).

Scliar-Cabral, L. (2013). *Sistema Scliar de alfabetização: fundamentos.* [*Scliar literacy system: fundamentals*] Florianópolis: Lili.

Stanovich, K. E. (1992). *Speculations on the causes and consequences of individual differences in early reading acquisition.* doi: http://dx.doi.org/10.1590/S0104-406020100003.

Torgesen, J. K. and Davis, C. (1996). Individual difference variables that predict response to training in phonological awareness. *Journal of Experimental Child Psychology*, 63(1), 1 - 21. Doi: 10.1590/S0104-40602010000300005.

Torgesen, J. K., Morgan, S. T. and Davis, C. (1992). Effects of two types of phonological awareness training on word learning in kindergarten children. *Journal of Educational psychology*, 84(3), 364. Doi:10.1037/0022-0663.84.3.364.

Wagner, R. K., Torgesen, J. K., Rashotte, C. A. and Pearson, N. A. (1999). *CTOPP examiner's manual*. PRO-ED, Austin, TX.

In: Dyslexia
Editors: Catia Giaconi et al.
ISBN: 978-1-53617-593-6
© 2020 Nova Science Publishers, Inc.

Chapter 3

TIER 2 RESPONSE TO INTERVENTION (RTI) MODEL: INTERVENTION WITH ALPHABETICAL PRINCIPLE AND METAPHONOLOGICAL SKILLS

Alexandra Beatriz Portes de Cerqueira César,
Melissa Pinotti Marguti and Simone Aparecida Capellini
Investigation Learning Disabilities Laboratory (LIDA), Department of Speech and Hearing Sciences, São Paulo State University "Júlio de Mesquita Filho" (UNESP), Marilia, São Paulo, Brazil

INTRODUCTION

Phonological awareness refers to the perception of parts of oral language such as rhymes, syllables and phonemes and how these parts combine in order to form new words. It is recognized in the literature that understanding the phonological organization of oral language, called phonological awareness, supports the acquisition of the alphabetic principle and, consequently, the ability to read (Cunningham & Carroll, 2012).

Likewise, the alphabetic principle – the knowledge that phonemes can be represented by letters - is a necessary condition for the complete mastery of reading in an alphabetic writing system, since the more automatic the access to letter names and the sounds they represent is, the most satisfying will be the decoding of words (Nicolau & Navas, 2015).

Phonological intervention, with the work of metaphonological skills, alphabet knowledge and grapheme-phoneme correspondence, when applied collectively, can play an important role in the identification of students with dyslexia, as these less intensive interventions are of a preventive and remediative nature, implementing relatively brief sessions of interventions to allow students to track reading performance and to identify students with more significant difficulties that may require more extensive and intensive interventions (Wanzek et al., 2013; Aravena et al., 2016).

The identification of students at risk for the development of reading at the beginning of literacy allows the intervention before manifestation of significant impairments in learning, so that with the intervention, the student can have a better prognosis in relation to their class group (Navas, 2011).

Due to the importance of early identification, this study is based on the hypothesis that a Collective Program of Phonological Remediation and Alphabetical Principle for students in early literacy, intervening in metaphonological skills, namely alphabet knowledge and grapheme-phoneme correspondence could identify students with dyslexia maximizing educational opportunities for all students as a way of prevention.

This study aimed to develop a second-tier intervention response (RTI) program to develop the alphabetic principle and metaphonological skills for students at risk for dyslexia and to verify the clinical significance of the elaborate collective program.

METHODS

This study was conducted after approval by the Research Ethics Committee of the Faculty of Philosophy and Sciences of São Paulo State University "Júlio de Mesquita Filho" (UNESP), Marilia, São Paulo, Brazil, under the number CAEE No. 0663/2013.

Elaboration of the Collective Intervention Program for the Development of Metaphonological Skills and Alphabetic Principle

The Elaboration of the Intervention Response Program (RTI) was developed based on the literature survey based on the following aspects:

1) Review of the literature on metaphonological and alphabetic principle strategies used in interventional procedures;
2) Description of tasks with the described objectives;
3) Duration of tasks and
4) Number of sessions in the programs.

Linguistic stimuli (real words) and visual stimuli (figures) were selected to be used in the activities that were elaborated, based on the alphabetic writing system. These stimuli were selected from the bank of pictures and words grouped by series, length and frequency, extracted from the texts contained in the Portuguese Language textbooks, from the Investigation Learning Disabilities Laboratory (LIDA) of the Faculty of Philosophy and Science of UNESP.

The Intervention Response Program (RTI) developed for this study consisted of twelve phonological tests, and these tasks were developed to be worked on in six sessions: Knowledge of the letter-sound;

Knowledge of syllable; Syllable segmentation; Phonemic segmentation; Syllable addition; Phonemic addition; Syllable subtraction; Phonemic subtraction; Syllable substitution; Phonemic substitution; Syllable Combination and Phonemic Combination.

Collective Intervention Program Activity

The program was designed from 8 individual sessions, with an initial individual session used for pre-testing, six 50-minute collective sessions for Intervention and a final individual session for post-testing.

Thus, the sessions were constituted as follows:

- *Session 1:* Knowledge of letter-sound and Knowledge of syllable;
- *Session 2:* Knowledge of letter-sound and Knowledge of syllable;
- *Session 3:* Syllable and phonemic segmentation, Syllabic and phonemic addition, Syllabic and phonemic subtraction;
- *Session 4:* Syllabic and phonemic segmentation, Syllabic and phonemic addition, Syllabic and phonemic subtraction;
- *Session 5:* Syllable and phonemic substitution and Syllable and phonemic combination;
- *Session 6:* Syllable and Phonemic Substitution and Syllable and Phonemic Combination.

Pilot Study

After the program elaboration, a pilot study was conducted with five subjects identified as at risk for dyslexia from the first to the second year of elementary school, with ages from 6 years to 7 years and

11 months of age in order to verify the existence of possible inconsistencies in the elaborated program; observe how the subjects performed the tasks according to the degree of difficulty elaborated, the material handling, the time of accomplishment of each session and to verify the index of reliable change and clinical significance of the results in situation of pre and post testing.

The criteria for selecting the students in this study were: Signing of the free and informed consent form; lack of history of speech, language, education or psychopedagogic intervention; and absence of attention deficit verified through neuropsychological evaluation.

All individuals who participated in this study were submitted the Early Identification Protocol for Reading Problems - IPPL (Capellini, César & Germano, 2017) as pre-testing and post-testing.

The results of the Pilot Study were analyzed using the JT Method (Jacobson & Truax, 1991; Del prette & del prette, 2008) for single case analysis.

The JT Method provides a comparative analysis between pre and post intervention scores in order to establish whether the differences between them represent reliable changes and are clinically relevant, thus allowing to verify the therapeutic efficacy by measuring clinical significance.

This method therefore implies two complementary processes, namely: (a) calculation of the reliability of changes occurring between the pre and post-intervention assessment, described in terms of a Reliable Change Index (BMI); and (b) analysis of the clinical significance of these changes. The difference is calculated based on the difference between pre and post-test divided by the standard error of the difference. Thus, the change from pre to post-test can be reliable positive (when there is improvement); reliable negative (when it gets worse); with clinical significance (which makes or will make a difference in the clinical setting); or absence of change.

RESULTS

The performance of the subjects of this study will be presented in the tests of the Early Identification of Reading Problems - IPPL (Capellini, César, & Germano, 2017). These tests were: alphabet knowledge, rhyme production, rhyme identification, syllable segmentation, word production from the given phoneme, phonemic synthesis, phonemic analysis, initial sound identification, phonological working memory, fast automatic naming, silent reading, reading words and pseudo words and understanding sentences from figures.

Table 1 shows the reliability of change in IPPL tests in the Pilot Study subjects.

Table 1. Reliability of change in IPPL tests in Pilot Study subjects

Subjects	KA	RP	RI	SS	WPP	PS	PA	IPI	PWM	SR	RAN	RWPW	CSF
1	-	-	RPC	RPC	RPC	RPC	RPC	RPC	-	RPC	-	RPC	
2	-	-	RPC	RPC	RPC	RPC	RPC	RPC	-	RPC	-	-	
3	RPC	-	-	-	-	-	-	-	-	-	-	-	
4	RPC	-	-	-	-	-	RPC	-	-	-	-	RPC	

Caption: KA: knowledge of the alphabet; RP: rhyme production; RI: Rhyme identification; SS: syllable segmentation; WPP: word production from given phoneme; PS: phonemic synthesis; PA: phonemic analysis; IPI: initial phoneme identification; PWM: phonological working memory; SR: silent reading; RAN: rapid automatized naming; RWPW: reading words and pseudo words; CSF: comprehension of sentences from figures; RPC: reliable positive change.

The subjects S1 and S2 are above the upper diagonal tracing, that is, they presented improvement that can be attributed to the intervention in the rhyme identification, syllable synthesis, word production from the given phoneme, phonemic synthesis, phonemic analysis, identifying of initial phoneme, silent reading and reading of words and pseudo words. In addition to being above the upper horizontal line and to the left of the vertical line, they showed improvement in clinical status, moving to the functional population for such skills.

Subject S4 showed improvement that can be attributed to the intervention in the knowledge skills of the alphabet, phonemic analysis and reading of words and pseudo words. In addition, he presented improvement in clinical status, moving to the functional population for these skills.

Subject S3 showed improvement that can be attributed to the intervention in the ability to know the alphabet.

DISCUSSION

Using national and international literature (Almeida, 2014; Andrade, Prado, Capellini, 2011; Carney & Stiefel, 2008; Fletcher & Vaughn, 2010; Machado & Capellini, 2014; Machado, Silva & Capellini, 2015; Pinheiro, Correa & Mousinho, 2012; Van Viersen et al., 2015; Vaughn et al., 2010; Wanzek & Vaughn, 2011), we analyze studies that used phonological intervention programs as part of the second-tier intervention response model for the work of the skills selected in the present study, covering the age range of six years and eleven months to seven years and eleven months of age.

During the analysis it was found that, in the national literature (Almeida, 2014; Andrade, Prado & Capellini, 2011; Machado & Capellini, 2014; Machado, Silva & Capellini, 2015; Pinheiro, Correa & Mousinho, 2012), there are few programs or strategies that use phonological intervention and grapheme-phoneme correspondence being performed collectively for this age group, which are or are not part of the intervention response model (RTI).

In contrast, in the international literature, not only there are a greater number of articles and works described for this age group and skills, but also references to programs are found in all layers of the RTI, both individually and collectively that work both the alphabetic principle and metaphonological skills geared for clinical and educational environment (Carney & Stiefel, 2008; Fletcher & Vaughn, 2010; Van Viersen et al., 2015; Vaughn et al., 2010; Wanzek & Vaughn, 2011). The American National Literacy Panel (NELP, 2010) reported that the metaphonological ability worked in the early literacy phase was considered as one of the most robust predictors of reading decoding, reading comprehension, and spelling skills. Therefore, internationally, it is imperative to identify effective models of emerging literacy intervention, allowing all students to have the opportunity to become good readers.

From this study it was possible to verify expressive improvement in the students' performance in the post-test in relation to the pre-test, evidenced in the tests of knowledge of the alphabet (CA), syllable segmentation (SS), word production from the given phoneme (PPF), phonemic synthesis (SF), phonemic analysis (AF), identification of the initial sound of the word (ISI), silent reading (LS) and reading of words and pseudo words (LPPP), favoring mainly the phonological skills considered important for the development of reading and writing in an alphabetic writing system (Capellini, 2012), after being submitted to the Collective Intervention Program Program for the development of metaphonological skills and alphabetic principle, elaborated in this study.

CONCLUSION

It was possible to elaborate a second layer intervention response program (RTI) to develop the alphabetic principle and metaphonological skills, based on the literature specialized in the area, so that this second layer intervention response study (RTI) enables the detection, early identification and intervention in at-risk students, so that dyslexia is diagnosed early in students who are in the early stages of literacy.

REFERENCES

Andrade, O. V., Andrade, P. E., & Capellini, S. A. (2014). Characterization of the cognitive-linguistic profile of students with reading and writing difficulties. *Psychology: Research and Review*, 358-367.

Andrade, O. V., Andrade, P. E., & Capellini, S. A. (2015). Collective screening tools for early identification of dyslexia. *Frontiers in psychology*, 5, 1581.

Andrade, O. V., Prado, P. S. T., & Capellini, S. A. (2011). Development of pedagogical tools to identify students at risk for dyslexia. *Psychopedagogy*, 14-28.

Aravena, S., Tijms, J., Snellings, P., & van der Molen, M. W. (2016). Predicting responsiveness to intervention in dyslexia using dynamic assessment. *Learning and Individual Differences, 49,* 209-215.

Bollman, K. A., Silberglitt, B., & Gibbons, K. A. (2007). The St. Croix River education district model: Incorporating systems-level organization and a multi-tiered problem-solving process for intervention delivery. *In: Handbook of response to intervention.* Springer, Boston, MA. 319-330.

Borges, L. K. S. *Effectiveness of the phonological remediation program in students with difficulties in learning to read and write in private teaching.* Scientific research (FAPESP 04/15556-5). Faculty of Philosophy and Science. 120 f. Marília, 2002.

Capellini, S. A., Cerqueira-César, A. B. P., & Germano, G. D. (2015). Early Identification of Reading Problems: Preliminary Study with Students of 1st Grade. *Procedia-Social and Behavioral Sciences*, 174, 1351-1355.

Capellini, S. A., Cerqueira César, A. B. P., & Germano, G. D. (2017). *Protocol for Early Identification of Reading Problems – IPPL.* Ribeirão Preto: BookToy.

Capovilla, A. G. S., & Capovilla, F. C. (2000). Effects of phonological awareness training in children with low socioeconomic status. *Psychology: Research and Review*, 13(1), 1- 28.

Caravolas, M., Lervåg, A., Mousikou, P., Efrim, C., Litavský, M., Onochie-Quintanilla, E., ... & Seidlová-Málková, G. (2012). Common patterns of prediction of literacy development in different alphabetic orthographies. *Psychological science*, 23(6), 678-686.

Cardoso, R. K. O. A., & Capellini, S. A. (2009). Effectiveness of the phonological awareness intervention program in schoolchildren at risk for dyslexia. *Psychopedagogy*, 26(81), 367-375.

Carney, K. J., & Stiefel, G. S. (2008). Long-Term Results of a Problem-Solving Approach to Response to Intervention: Discussion and Implications. *Learning Disabilities: A Contemporary Journal*, 6(2), 61-75.

Cerqueira César, A. B. P., Capellini, S. A., & Germano, G. D. (2018). *Phonological Remediation Program for students at risk for dyslexia - PROF-RD*. Ribeirão Preto, São Paulo: BookToy.

Del Prette, Z. A. P., & Del Prette, A. (2008). Clinical significance and reliable change in the assessment of psychological interventions. *Psychology: theory and research*, 24(4), 497-505.

Fukuda, M. T. M., & Capellini, S. A. (2012). Phonological intervention program associated with grapheme-phoneme correspondence in students at risk for dyslexia. *Psychology: Research and Review*, 783-790.

Fletcher, J. M., & Vaughn, S. (2009). Response to intervention: Preventing and remediating academic difficulties. *Child development perspectives*, 3(1), 30-37.

Germano, G. D., César, A. B. P. C., & Capellini, S. A. (2017). Screening Protocol for Early Identification of Brazilian Children at Risk for Dyslexia. *Frontiers in psychology*, 8, 1763.

Graminha, S. S. V., Machado, V. L. S., Francischini, E. L., & Befi, V. M. (1987). Use of a gradual syllable discrimination training procedure in children with reading and writing difficulties. *Brazilian Archives of Psychology, 39*(1), 84-94.

Griffiths, Y., & Stuart, M. (2013). Reviewing evidence-based practice for pupils with dyslexia and literacy difficulties. *Journal of Research in Reading,* 36(1), 96-116.

Harris, K. R., Graham, S., & Adkins, M. (2015). Practice-based professional development and self-regulated strategy development for Tier 2, at-risk writers in second grade. *Contemporary Educational Psychology,* 40, 5-16.

Jacobson, N. S., Truax, P. (1991). Clinical significance: a statistical approach to defining meaningful change in psychotherapy research. *Journal of consulting and clinical psychology,* 59(1), 12.

Fusco, N., Germano, G. D., & Capellini, S. A. (2015). Effectiveness of a perceptual-visual-motor intervention program for students with dyslexia. *CoDAS,* 27(2), 128-134.

Fukuda, M. T. M., & Capellini, S. A. (2012). Phonological intervention program associated with grapheme-phoneme correspondence in students at risk for dyslexia. *Psychology: Research and Review,* 783-790.

Machado, A. C., & Almeida, M. A. (2012). Performance in reading tasks using the rti model: response to intervention in public school students. *Psychopedagogy,* 29(89), 208-214.

Machado, A. C., & Almeida, M. A. (2014). The RTI-Response to intervention model as an inclusive proposal for students with reading and writing difficulties. *Psychopedagogy,* 31(95), 130-143.

Machado, A. C., & Capellini, S. A. (2014). Reading and writing tutoring based on the ITN model – response to intervention in children with developmental dyslexia. *CEFAC,* 1161-1167.

Moll, K., Ramus, F., Bartling, J., Bruder, J., Kunze, S., Neuhoff, N., ... & Tóth, D. (2014). Cognitive mechanisms underlying reading and spelling development in five European orthographies. *Learning and Instruction,* 29, 65-77.

Navas, A. L. G. P. (2011). Why prevention is better than cure when it comes to learning disabilities. In: Alves LM, Mousinho R & Capellini S (Org). Dyslexia: new themes, new perspectives. *Rio de Janeiro: Wak Publishing company.* 2011, v I. P. 41-53.

Nicolau, C. C., & Navas, A. L. G. P. (2015). Assessment of the predictive skills of reading success in children from 1st and 2nd years of elementary school. *CEFAC*, 17(3), 917-926.

Pape-Neumann, J., van Ermingen-Marbach, M., Grande, M., Willmes, K., & Heim, S. (2015). The role of phonological awareness in treatments of dyslexic primary school children. *Acta Neurobiol. Exp.*, 75, 80-106.

Pinheiro, L., Correa, J., & Mousinho, R. (2012). The effectiveness of speech therapy remediation strategies in the assessment of learning difficulties. *Psychopedagogy*, 29(89), 215-225.

Cavalheiro, L. G., Santos, M. D., & Martinez, P. C. (2010). Influence of phonological awareness on reading acquisition. *CEFAC*, 12(6), 1009-1016.

Schickedanz, J. A., & McGee, L. M. (2010). The NELP report on shared story reading interventions (Chapter 4) extending the story. *Educational Researcher*, 39(4), 323-329.

Silva, C., & Capellini, S. A. (2015). Effectiveness of a phonological intervention program in students at risk for dyslexia. *CEFAC*, 1827-1837.

Silva, C., & Capellini, S. A. (2010). Effectiveness of the phonological and reading remediation program on learning disabilities. *Pró-fono*, 22(2), 131-139.

Snowling, M. J., & Hulme, C. (2012). Annual Research Review: The nature and classification of reading disorders–a commentary on proposals for DSM-5. *Journal of Child Psychology and Psychiatry*, 53(5), 593-607.

Teubal, E., & Dockrell, J. E. (2005). Children's developing numerical notations: The impact of input display, numerical size and operational complexity. *Learning and Instruction*, 15(3), 257-280.

Torgesen, J. K., & Davis, C. (1996). Individual difference variables that predict response to training in phonological awareness. *Journal of Experimental Child Psychology*, 63(1), 1-21.

Van Viersen, S., de Bree, E. H., Zee, M., Maassen, B., Van Der Leij, A., & de Jong, P. F. (2018). Pathways into literacy: The role of early oral language abilities and family risk for dyslexia. *Psychological science*, 29(3), 418-428.

Vaughn, S., Cirino, P. T., Wanzek, J., Wexler, J., Fletcher, J. M., Denton, C. D., ... & Francis, D. J. (2010). Response to intervention for middle school students with reading difficulties: Effects of a primary and secondary intervention. *School Psychology Review*, 39(1), 3.

Vaughn, S., Wanzek, J. (2014). Intensive interventions in reading for students with reading disabilities: Meaningful impacts. *Learning Disabilities Research & Practice*, 29(2), 46-53.

Vellutino, F. R., Fletcher, J. M., Snowling, M. J., & Scanlon, D. M. (2004). Specific reading disability (dyslexia): What have we learned in the past four decades? *Journal of child psychology and psychiatry*, 45(1), 2-40.

Wanzek, J., & Vaughn, S. (2011). Is a three-tier reading intervention model associated with reduced placement in special education? *Remedial and Special Education*, 32(2), 167-175.

Wanzek, J., Vaughn, S., Scammacca, N. K., Metz, K., Murray, C. S., Roberts, G., & Danielson, L. (2013). Extensive reading interventions for students with reading difficulties after grade 3. *Review of Educational Research*, 83(2), 163-195.

In: Dyslexia
Editors: Catia Giaconi et al.
ISBN: 978-1-53617-593-6
© 2020 Nova Science Publishers, Inc.

Chapter 4

ANALYSIS OF THE CLINICAL SIGNIFICANCE OF STUDENTS WITH DYSLEXIA IN READING PROCESS EVALUATION

Isabela Pires Metzner and Simone Aparecida Capellini
Investigation Learning Disabilities Laboratory (LIDA), Department of Speech and Hearing Sciences, São Paulo State University "Júlio de Mesquita Filho" (UNESP), Marilia, São Paulo, Brazil

INTRODUCTION

Dyslexia refers to differences in individual processing, often characterized by the difficulties presented at the beginning of literacy, compromising the acquisition of reading, writing, and spelling. Cognitive, phonological and/or visual processes may also fail (Reid, 2016).

Students with dyslexia have difficulty incorrect reading fluency and decoding ability, altered child discrimination, phonological awareness, and short-term memory limitation. They may also have problems with long-term verbal memory due to the difficulty of forming Mexico for storage, with consequent impairment in reading irregular, infrequent words, pseudowords, increased vocabulary and reading of reading material (Oliveira & Cardoso, 2012).

To perform activities such as reading isolated words or text, it is necessary a refined visual processing of the graphic signals to perform a textual scan to identify the constituent parts of the word, and it is necessary to consider that this visual processing is related to the linguistic processing of reading, which performs the identification of the word through the process of phonological decoding. Such a process allows the conversion of graphic signals into phonological representations. Children with attentional or information processing failures will have difficulty triggering refined visual processing, which will compromise the phonological access required for reading and writing an alphabetic system (Cardo, Servera, Vida, De Azua & Redondo, 2011; Capellini, Ferreira, Salgado & Ciasca, 2007).

Reading may occur through a process involving phonological mediation (phonological route) or through the direct visual process (lexical route). Reading through the phonological route depends on the use of knowledge of the rules of conversion between grapheme and phoneme so that the construction of the word pronunciation can be performed. Reading by the lexical route depends on prior knowledge of a word and memorization in the visual word recognition system, and on the retrieval of its meaning and pronunciation by direct addressing to the lexicon, such pronunciation being obtained as a whole. Both pathways are complementary and used in different measures during reading (Pinheiro, Lúcio & Silva, 2009; Pinheiro & Capellini, 2010).

For competent reading, the word must be recognized quickly and accurately. This rapid identification occurs due to the formation of the mental lexicon, in which familiar and high-frequency words are visually recognized, while the identification of new and low-frequency words depends on phonological strategies, in which the reader associates the letters to sounds (Roman, Kirby, Parrila, Wade-Woolley & Deacon, 2009).

This chapter's purpose to analyze the clinical significance of subjects with developmental dyslexia in the evaluation of reading processes.

METHOD

This study was conducted after approval by the Research Ethics Committee of the Faculty of Philosophy and Sciences of São Paulo State University "Júlio de Mesquita Filho" (UNESP), Marilia, São Paulo, Brazil, under the number CAEE No. 5873.1316.6.00005406.

Ten students with interdisciplinary diagnosis of Developmental Dyslexia participated in this study by an interdisciplinary team composed by speech, neurological, pedagogical and neuropsychological assessment of the Investigation Learning Disabilities Laboratory (LIDA), with ages between 8 and 11 years and 11 months, of both sexes, from the third to the fifth grade of elementary school in a city in the interior of São Paulo.

Eleven students were submitted to the Reading Process Assessment - PROLEC (Capellini, 2010) individually in a 50-minute session. This evaluation consists of four blocks distributed for the evaluation of four reading processes, as described below:

— *1st Process:* identification of letters- composed of two tests designed to measure the ability of students to identify letters and their respective sounds. The sound and letter identification test aim to verify the ability of the student to name the letters and the sound that represents them. The proof of equal and different words and pseudowords aims to verify the ability of the student to identify, discriminate and recognize real and invented words as being the same/different.

— *2nd Process:* lexical processes; composed of four tests to verify the functioning of the two-word recognition routes and their subprocesses. In lexical decision testing, the student must recognize only real words in a list of real and invented words regardless of whether or not they can read them. In the word reading, pseudoword reading and word and pseudoword tests, the objective is to compare the development of word recognition routes, and the student must perform the reading of real words and invented words, and in the first test it was The ability of the student to read real words and, in the second, the ability to read invented words of different syllable complexities, divided into CCV, VC, CVC, CVV, CCVC, and CVVC. In the third test, the objective is to analyze the degree of development that the student achieved with the use of phonological and lexical routes for reading. For this, we used words and pseudowords belonging to six categories: short high-frequency words, long high-frequency words, short low-frequency words, long low-frequency words, short pseudowords, and long pseudowords.

— *3rd Process:* syntactic processes; composed of two tests. In the test of grammatical structures, it is verified the ability of the student to process different types of grammatical structures and to prove the difficulty that can be produced when using different syntactic structures, namely: active voice, passive voice, and focused complement. In the test of punctuation marks, it is observed the ability of the student to use punctuation marks in a small text.

— *4th Process:* semantic processes; composed of two tests. In the Prayer Comprehension test, the goal is to assess whether the student is able to extract the meaning of simple prayers. In the text comprehension test, the objective is to investigate if the student is able to extract the meaning and integrate it with their knowledge.

The analysis of the results was performed using the JT Method which provides a comparative analysis between pre and post-intervention scores in order to decide if the differences between them represent reliable changes and if they are clinically relevant.

Data analysis using the JT Method, therefore, implies two complementary processes: (a) calculating the reliability of changes between scores, described in terms of a Reliable Change Index (BMI); and (b) analysis of the clinical significance of these changes. Based on quantitative indicators, these two processes can be graphically represented. (Del prette; Del prette, 2008).

RESULTS

In Graph 1, five students diagnosed with dyslexia underperformed and five students diagnosed with dyslexia presented an average performance in the test Name or sound of letters.

In Graph 2, three students diagnosed with dyslexia underperformed and seven students diagnosed with dyslexia presented an average performance on the test Equal or different.

In Graph 3, two students diagnosed with dyslexia underperformed and eight students diagnosed with dyslexia presented an average performance on the lexical decision test.

In Graph 4, five students diagnosed with Dyslexia underperformed and five students diagnosed with Dyslexia presented an average performance on the Word Reading test.

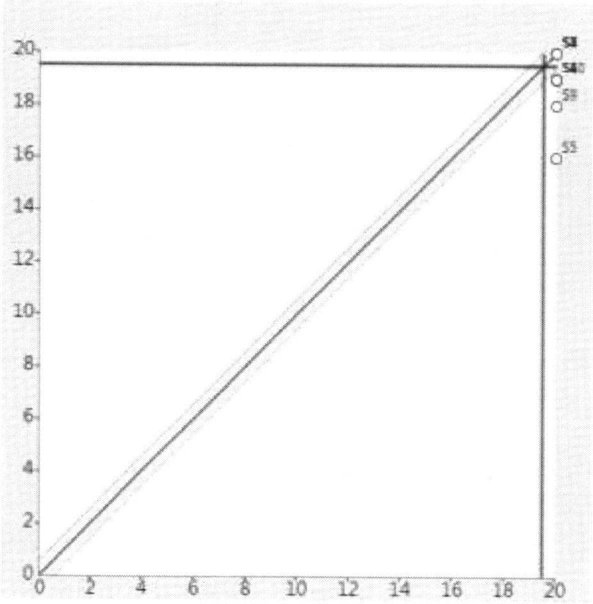

Graph 1. Clinical significance of students with dyslexia in the Name test or letter sound.

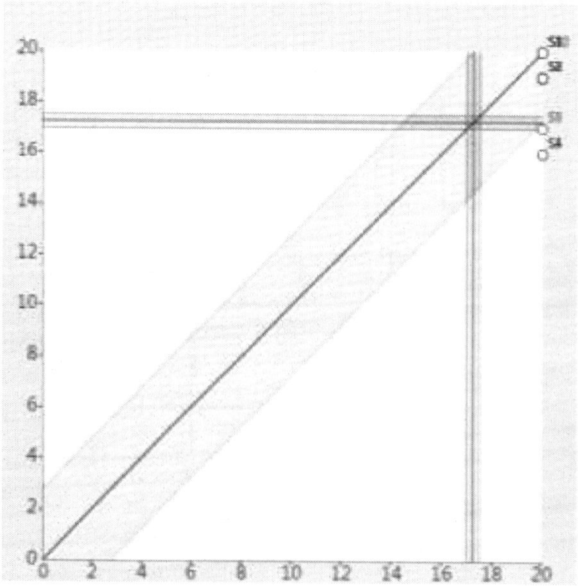

Graph 2. Clinical significance of students with dyslexia in the test Equal or different.

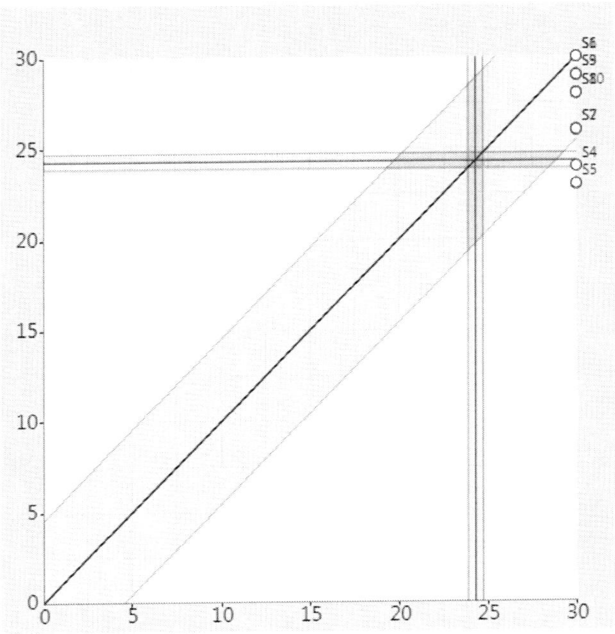

Graph 3. Clinical significance of students with dyslexia in the lexical decision test.

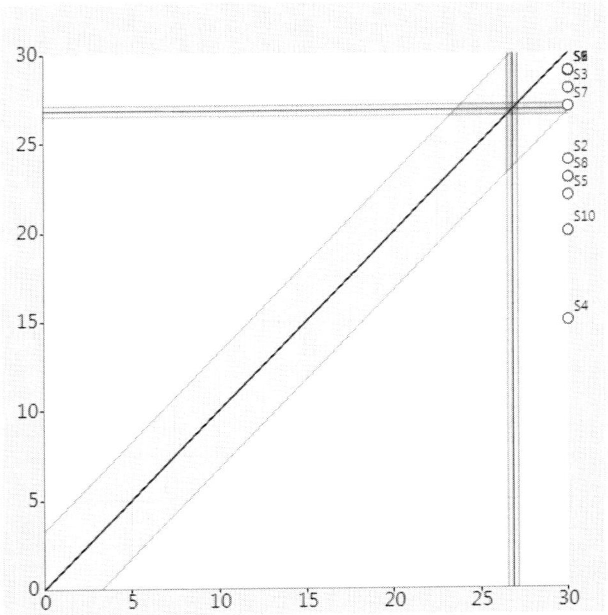

Graph 4. Clinical significance of students with dyslexia in the test Word reading.

In Graph 5, five students diagnosed with dyslexia underperformed and five students diagnosed with dyslexia presented an average performance on the test Pseudoword reading.

In Graph 6, nine students diagnosed with dyslexia underperformed and one student diagnosed with dyslexia presented an average performance in the test Frequent word reading.

In Graph 7, five students diagnosed with Dyslexia underperformed and five students diagnosed with Dyslexia showed an average performance on the test Reading of infrequent words.

In Graph 8, six students diagnosed with dyslexia underperformed and four students diagnosed with dyslexia presented an average performance on the test Pseudoword reading.

In Graph 9, eight students diagnosed with dyslexia underperformed and two students diagnosed with dyslexia presented an average performance on the Grammatical Structures test.

Graph 5. Clinical significance of students with dyslexia in the test Pseudoword reading.

Analysis of the Clinical Significance of Students ... 51

Graph 6. Clinical significance of students with dyslexia in the test Frequent word reading.

Graph 7. Clinical significance of students with dyslexia in the test Reading of infrequent words.

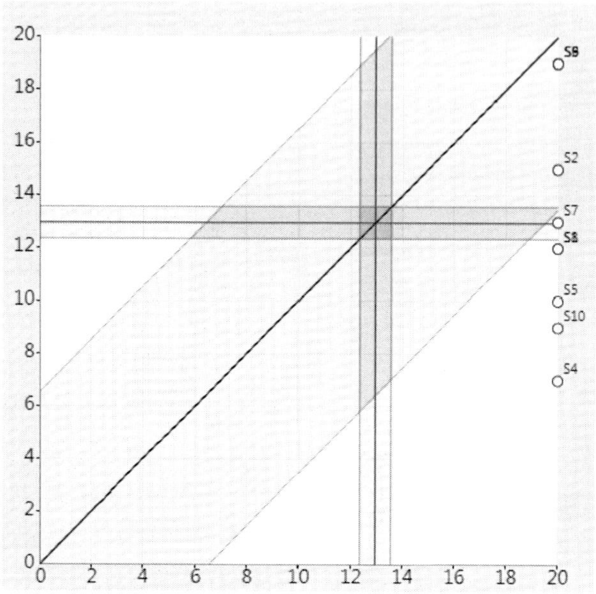

Graph 8. Clinical significance of students with dyslexia in the test Pseudoword reading.

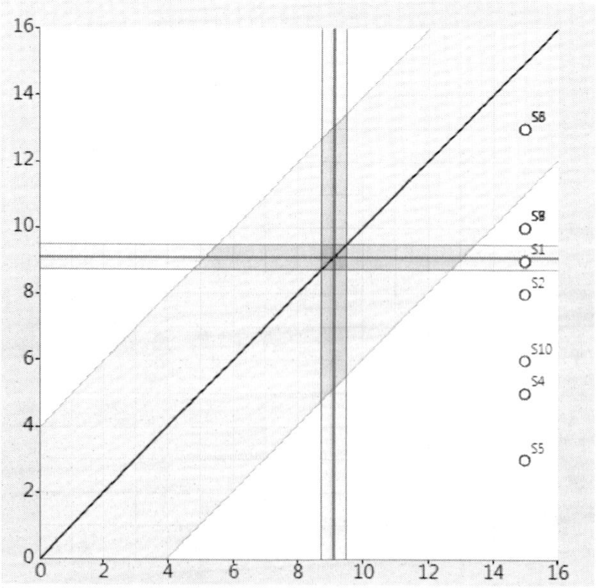

Graph 9. Clinical significance of students with dyslexia in the test Grammatical structures.

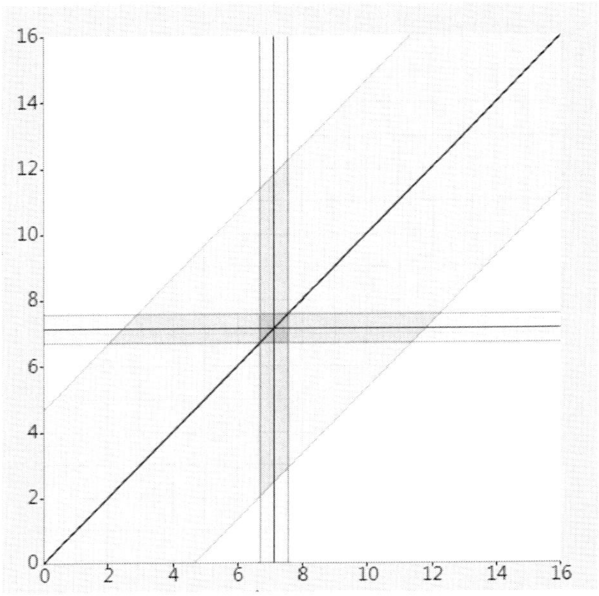

Graph 10. Clinical significance of students with dyslexia in the test Punctuation marks.

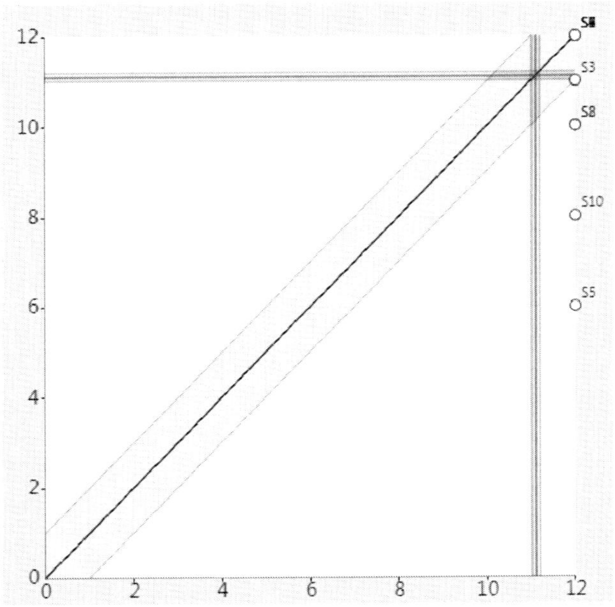

Graph 11. Clinical significance of students with dyslexia in the test Understanding prayers.

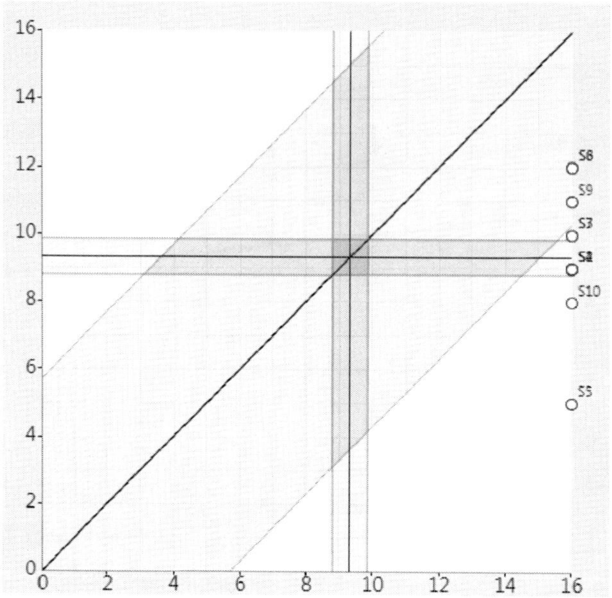

Graph 12. Clinical significance of students with dyslexia in the test Text comprehension.

In Graph 10, ten students diagnosed with Dyslexia performed on average on the Grammatical Structures test.

In Graph 11, five students diagnosed with dyslexia underperformed and five students diagnosed with dyslexia presented an average performance on the Grammatical Structures test.

In Graph 12, seven students diagnosed with dyslexia underperformed and three students diagnosed with dyslexia presented an average performance on the Grammatical Structures test.

DISCUSSION

According to the results obtained in this study, it is possible to verify that the students with Dyslexia presented underperformance in the tests that measure the performance in letter identification, lexical process, semantic process and syntactic process. This result corroborates study (Oliveira & Cardoso, 2012) that stated that dyslexics present poor performance in lexical, syntactic and semantic processes.

Our findings regarding the performance of dyslexic students in this study corroborated studies in countries that have Spanish as the official language (Escribano, 2007; Bednarek, Saldana & García, 2009; Jimenéz, Rodrigués & Ramírez, 2009; Aguilar, Navarro, Menachi & Alcale, 2010) that used PROLEC to evaluate reading processes in students with dyslexia. Difficulties were identified in tasks that require the use of phonological skills, which are necessary for reading.

Students with developmental dyslexia had poor performance in the tests of Name or sound of letters and grammatical structures, this result corroborates a study (Pennala et al., 2010) that states that dyslexics present difficulties in grapheme-phoneme conversion, which impairs the development of reading, discrimination of sounds and verbal memory. As a limitation of this study, it is possible to point out that the performance of students with developmental dyslexia in these tests may be a consequence of the selection of subjects, since the selection of subjects who were part of the sample of this study did not follow inclusion criteria for dyslexia subtypes.

Conclusion

The findings of this study showed that subjects with Developmental Dyslexia performed below expectations in the letter identification, lexical, syntactic and semantic processes.

References

Aguilar, VM, Navarro GJI, Menacho JI, Alcale CC, Marchena Consejeto E, Ramiro Olivier P. Speed of naming and phonological awareness in the initial learning of reading. *Psychothema.* 2010;22(3):436-42. Available in: dialnet.unirioja.es/servlet/Article?codigo=3258251

Bednarek, D, Saldaña D, García I. Visual versus phonological abilities in Spanish dyslexic boys and girls. *Brain and Cognition.* 2009;70 (3):273-8. Available in: 10.1016/j.bandc.2009.02.010.

Cardo, E, Servera M, Vidal C, De Azua B, Redondo M. Influence of the different diagnostic criteria and culture in the prevalence of attention deficit hyperactivity disorder. *Neurology journals.* 2011; 52 (1): 109-17. Available in: 10.33588/rn. 52S01.2010793.

Capellini, SA. PROLEC: Evidence of evaluation of reading processes. São Paulo: *Psychologist's House.* 2010.

Capellini, SA, Ferreira T, Salgado C, Ciasca SM. Performance of schoolchildren who are good readers, with dyslexia and with attention deficit hyperactivity disorder in rapid automatic naming. *Revista Sociedade Brasileira Fonoaudiologia* 2007; 12 (2): 114-119. Available in: 10.1590/S1516-80342007000200008.

Escribano, CL. Evaluation of the double-deficit hypothesis subtype classification of reader in Spanish. *Journal of Learning Disabilities.* 2007;40(4):319-30. Available in: 10.1177/00222194070400040301.

Jiménez, JE, Rodríguez C, Ramírez G. Spanish developmental dyslexia. Prevalence, cognitive profile, and home literacy experiences. *Journal of Experimental Child Psychology.* 2009;103(2):167-85. Available in: 10.1016/j. jecp.2009.02.004.

Pennala, Rl, Eklund K, Hämäläinen J, Richardson U, Martin M, Leiwo M, Leppänen PH, Lyytinen H. Perception of phonemic length and its relation to reading andspelling skills in children with family risk for dyslexia in the first three grades of school. *Journal of speech and hearing research.* 2010; 53(3):710-24. Available in: 10.1044/1092-4388(2009/08-0133).

Pinheiro, AMV, Lúcio PS, Silva DMR. Cognitive reading evaluation: the effect of grapheme-phoneme and phoneme-grapheme regularity on reading aloud of isolated words in Brazilian Portuguese. *Journal* of *Psychology-Theory and Practice*. 2009; 10 (2). Available in: http://pepsic.bvsalud.org/scielo.php?script=sci_arttext&pid=S1516-36872008000200002.

Pinheiro, FH, Capellini SA. Auditory training in students with learning disabilities. *Pro-Phono*.2010;22(1):49-54. Available in: 10.1590/S0104 56872010000100010.

Reid, G. (2016). Dyslexia: *A practitioner's handbook*. John Wiley & Sons.

In: Dyslexia
Editors: Catia Giaconi et al.
ISBN: 978-1-53617-593-6
© 2020 Nova Science Publishers, Inc.

Chapter 5

CLINICAL SIGNIFICANCE OF TEXT READING COMPREHENSION AFTER REMEDIATION WITH RAPID NAMING AND READING

Bianca dos Santos and Simone Aparecida Capellini
Investigation Learning Disabilities Laboratory (LIDA),
Department of Speech and Hearing Sciences,
São Paulo State University "Júlio de Mesquita Filho"
(UNESP), Marilia, São Paulo, Brazil

INTRODUCTION

Dyslexia refers to differences in individual processing, often characterized by the difficulties presented at the beginning of literacy, which undermines the acquisition of reading, writing and spelling. Cognitive, phonological and/or visual processes may also present flaws (Reid 2016).

The difficulties that students with Developmental Dyslexia present result from a deficit that these students face in phonological processing, which is generally below expectations when compared to other cognitive abilities. Thus, the student may show difficulty in textual comprehension and have reduced reading experience due to this disorder (International Dyslexia Association 2013).

The rapid automatized naming test is considered in the literature as a predictor of the development of reading and writing, especially for decoding skills, fluency and consequently reading comprehension. (Catts 2002; Christo and Davis 2008).

During the reading process, a refined visual processing of the graphic signals is necessary to perform a textual scan in order to identify the constituent parts of the word and, consequently, their fixation, coding and further comprehension. Such skill is therefore required as soon as the child begins literacy. However, we must consider that this visual processing is related to the linguistic processing of reading, which performs the identification of the word through the phonological decoding process, which is aided by phonological representations. This process allows the conversion of graphic signals into phonological representations (Capellini; Salgado and Ciascae 2007).

Studies (Capellini and Lanza 2010; Capellini and Conrado 2009) show that students with dyslexia, when compared to students who do not have reading alteration, tend to take longer to perform the rapid automatic naming test and that such ability can be regarded as a prerequisite for reading performance. Reading comprehension is extremely challenging for students with dyslexia and reading difficulties, as many teachers emphasize that reading comprehension is one of the key skills to be acquired for reading (Edmonds et al. 2009; Awada; Plana 2018).

At the end of the early years of literacy, according to Millán (2008), the fluency with which students read words can predict their level of reading comprehension. Thus, when comparing two students with the same prior knowledge, the same ability to store information and operate with the so-called discourse markers, the reader who has a reading ability considered faster than the other will probably perform higher success rates in understanding tasks.

Reading comprehension problems are known to be an obstacle to learning, as all school assignments, not only those of Portuguese, require students to read and extract the information they need for their school learning. Students with comprehension problems cannot perform these tasks and differ from their class group in their performance (Stothard 2004).

Reading comprehension skills are related to decoding skills, supported by separate skills which predict the variation in comprehension tasks performance, i.e., the ability to integrate text information, text structure knowledge and metacognitive monitoring and operational phonological memory (Kida; Chiari and Ávila 2010; Capellini; Santos and Uvo 2015). Thus, reading comprehension will depend on the individual's ability to decode and quickly recognize individual words, automatically and fluently; this ability to understanding can be greatly impaired when the student has some difficulty recognizing the words (Capellini; Santos and Uvo 2015).

According to Solé (1998) and Cunha and Capellini (2014), texts are classified into categories according to their structure, and may be descriptive, expository, narrative, descriptive and instructive-inductive. However, most research is based on discussing students' performance in understanding narrative or expository texts, such as this study, due to the fact that since their childhood there has been a greater exposure to these textual categories.

It is possible to verify the performance of students in reading comprehension through expository texts, because according to the authors (Escudero and León 2007; Cunha and Capellini 2014) these texts do not have organizational milestones so clear, differently from narrative texts.

This chapter´s purpose to present the clinical significance through the JT Method of performance of individuals with developmental dyslexia in reading comprehension after undergoing intervention with

Remediation with Rapid Automatized Naming and Reading (Santos and Capellini 2018).

METHOD

This study was conducted after approval by the Research Ethics Committee of the Faculty of Philosophy and Sciences of São Paulo State University "Júlio de Mesquita Filho" (UNESP), Marilia, São Paulo, Brazil, under the number CAAE 45213015.0.0000.5406.

To compose this study, 5 individuals from the 3rd to the 5th grade of Elementary School, from 9 years to 11 years and 11 months, diagnosed with Developmental Dyslexia participated;

All individuals submitted the Remediation with Rapid Automatized Naming Program and the pre and post-test situation. The parents signed the Informed Consent Form agreeing to participate in this study and the data collection was performed against the school shift.

Reading Remediation Program and Rapid Automatized Naming - PRONAR-LE

The Remediation Program with Rapid Automatized Naming - PRONAR-LE (Santos and Capellini 2018) aims to intervene with rapid temporal fusion in succession - necessary for rapid automatic naming and reading - thereby favoring possible improvement in decoding, accuracy, speed, fluency and consequently reading comprehension of students with learning difficulties and disorders.

The Program is divided into 6 sessions, so that every two sessions the boards are repeated. It is made up of four-syllable, single-syllable, four-syllable picture, word, pseudo word, and non-word picture, name, and pseudo word naming boards, so that with each session the complexity of both extension and syllable increase.

The students were in care for 5 weeks, so that the first and last weeks were used for pre and post-test. All subjects were submitted the following Protocol in pre- and post-testing moments:

Reading Comprehension Assessment Protocol - PROCOMLE (Cunha and Capellini 2014): This procedure consists of four texts: two narrative texts and two expository texts. The expository text (E1 "O Piolho") was used for this study, in order to verify the performance in the question types (literal and inferential question related to the microstructure and the macrostructure of the text), which can be used both collectively in the text in educational context, as in the individual form, in the clinical context.

In order to analyze the performance of the subjects who underwent the remediation program in pre and post-test situation, the JT method was used. This method provides a comparative analysis of pre- and post-intervention scores to decide whether differences between them represent reliable changes (BMI) and whether they are clinically relevant (SC) (Jacobson and Truax 1991; Del Prette and Del Prette 2008). Through this method it is possible to obtain descriptive dimensions of the individual's performance.

RESULTS

Table 1 will show the reliability of Change and Clinical Significance in reading comprehension through the text "O Piolho" in individuals with dyslexia.

According to Table 1, four subjects with dyslexia showed reliable positive change in reading comprehension, and two of those changes had clinical significance after undergoing the Remediation Program with Fast Automatic Naming and Reading.

Table 1. Reliability of Change and Clinical Significance in reading comprehension through the text E1 in subjects with Dyslexia

Subjects	E1	
1	MPC	-
2	MPC	SC
3	MPC	SC
4	-	-
5	MPC	

Caption: E: expository text; MPC: reliable positive change; SC: clinical significance.

DISCUSSION

Textual comprehension includes several interrelated cognitive processes; among them, basic readings processes, such as recognizing and extracting the meaning of printed words, are necessary requirements, although they are not the only ones sufficient for comprehension to occur. Successful textual comprehension requires high-level cognitive processes, such as the ability to make inferences, general language skills, memory skills, world knowledge, which together contribute to the construction of a macrostructural representation of the text (Salles and Parente 2002; Navas Pinto and Delissa 2009).

The Rapid Automatic Naming and Reading Remediation program enabled subjects to improve reading fluency and consequently reading automation, also improving reading comprehension, as reading fluency is essential for comprehension (Wolf and Denckla 2005).

The improvement in reading comprehension performance of students with developmental dyslexia can be attributed to the automation worked in the intervention through rapid automatic naming and reading, corroborating a study by Silva (2015) that showed that automatic naming correlates with reading, since both require proper word recognition and use of the contents of spelling and lexical processing.

According to authors (Fletcher, Lyons, Fuchs and Barnes 2009; Cunha and Capellini 2014), textual comprehension depends on one's ability to quickly decode and recognize isolated words fluently and quickly, so when the ability to read fluently is impaired, the subject also fails the ability to understand. Thus, the direct work with the speed of access to the lexicon and the rapid temporal fusion in succession, necessary for the task of performing the rapid automatic appointment, when worked in an intervention situation, has favored the developmental dyslexia students who manifest a deficit in reading comprehension.

According to studies (Silva 2017; Gray, Catts, Logan and Pentimonti 2017; Silva and Pereira 2019) reading comprehension plays a fundamental role in teaching-learning, for it is in the school phase that practices which require directly the teaching of reading and fluency to acquire new knowledge, being the difficulty in understanding one of the main ones, and it is necessary that these students first acquire the ability to decode and read fluently, demonstrated in this study that, when working the reading fluency, the students get better in reading comprehension consequently.

Fluency is a factor that can both facilitate and hinder comprehension, whether in oral or silent reading. Thus, we can state that the subjects with Dyslexia who underwent the intervention had an improvement in reading comprehension, because there was an improvement in reading fluency, since its absence is one of the factors that hinder the comprehension of the text read by subjects with some kind of difficulty (Miller and Schwanenflugel 2006).

One subject with developmental dyslexia showed no reliable positive change after undergoing the remediation program with rapid automatic naming and reading. This deficit in reading comprehension has great occurrence in subjects with developmental dyslexia, and deserves special attention as cited in the literature (Silva and Capellini, 2010; Oliveira; Cardoso and Capellini, 2012).

CONCLUSION

We can conclude that the intervention program with rapid automatic naming and reading proved to be effective and clinically significant in reading comprehension skills for students with Developmental Dyslexia, and it can be shown that this program can be used by speech and language pathologists as an instrument of intervention based on scientific evidence that helps the development of reading comprehension of these subjects.

REFERENCES

Awada, G. and Plana, M. G. C. (2018). Multiple Strategies Approach and EFL Reading Comprehension of Learners with Dyslexia: Teachers' Perceptions. *International Journal of Instruction*, 11(3), 463 - 476. DOI: 10.12973/iji.2018.11332a.

Capellini, S. A. and Conrado, T. L. B. C. (2009). Performance of students with and without learning difficulties in phonological awareness, rapid naming, reading and writing from the private education. *Rev. Cefac*, 11(2), 183 - 93. http://dx.doi.org/10.1590/S1516-18462009005000002.

Capellini, S. A. and Lanza, S. C. (2010). Students' performance in phonological awareness, rapid naming, reading, and writing. *Pró-Fono Revista de Atualização Científica,* 22(3), 239 - 244. http://dx.doi.org/10.1590/S0104-56872010000300014.

Capellini, S. A., Ferreira, T. L., Salgado, C. A and Ciasca, S. M. (2007). *Performance of good readers, students with dyslexia and attention deficit hyperactivity disorder in rapid automatized naming.* 12(20, 114 - 119. http://dx.doi.org/10.1590/ S1516-80342007000200008.

Capellini, S. A., Santos, B. and Uvo, M. F. C. (2015). Metalinguistic skills, reading and reading comprehension performance of students of the 5th grade. *Procedia-Social and Behavioral Sciences,* 174, 1346 - 1350. https://doi.org/10.1016/j.sbspro.2015.01.757.

Catts, H. W., Gillispie, M., Leonard, L. B., Kail, R. V. and Miller, C. A. (2002). The role of speed of processing, rapid naming, and phonological awareness in reading achievement. *Journal of learning disabilities,* 35(6), 510 - 525. https://doi.org/10.1177/00222194020350060301.

Christo, C. and Davis, J. (2008). Rapid naming and phonological processing as predictors of reading and spelling. *The California School Psychologist,* 13(1), 7 - 18. https://doi.org/10.1007/BF03340938.

Cunha, V. L. O. and Capellini, S. A. (2014*). Reading Comprehension Evaluation Protocol - PROCOMLE.* Booktoy: Ribeirão Preto.

Del Prette, Z. A. P. and Del Prette, A. (2008). *Clinical significance and reliable change in evaluating psychological interventions,* 24(4), 497 - 505. http://dx.doi.org/ 10.1590/S0102-37722008000400013.

Edmonds, M. S., Vaughn, S., Wexler, J., Reutebuch, C., Cable, A., Tackett, K. K. and Schnakenberg, J. W. (2009). A synthesis of reading interventions and effects on reading comprehension outcomes for older struggling readers. *Review of educational research,* 79(1), 262 - 300. https://doi.org/10.3102/0034654308325998.

Escudero, I. and León, J. A. (2007). Procesos inferenciales en la comprensión del discurso escrito: Infuencia de la estructura del texto en los procesos de comprensión. [Inferential processes in the comprehension of written discourse: Influence of the structure of the text in the comprehension processes.] *Revista signos,* 40(64), 311 - 336. http://dx.doi.org/10.4067/S0718-09342007000200003.

Fletcher, J. M., Lyons, G. R., Fuchs, L. S. and Barnes, M. A. (2009). *Learning Disabilities: from identification to intervention.* Porto Alegre: Artmed.

Gray, S., Catts, H., Logan, J. and Pentimonti, J. (2017). Oral language and listening comprehension: Same or different constructs? *Journal of Speech, Language, and Hearing Research,* 60, 1273 - 1284. doi:10.1044/2017_JSLHR-L-16-0039.

International Dyslexia Association. (2013). *Dyslexia in the classroom: what every teacher needs to know.* Recuperado de http://www.interdys.org/UnlockingDyslexiaPressRelease.htm [Consulta: 16 de outubro de 2019].

Jacobson, N. S. and Truax, P. (1991). *Clinical significance: a statistical approach to defining meaningful change in psychotherapy research,* 631 - 648. http://dx.doi.org/10.1037/10109-042.

Kida, A. D. S. B., Chiari, B. M. and de Ávila, C. R. B. (2010). Reading scale: proposal to assess reading skills. *Rev. Soc. Bras. Fonoaudiol.,* 15(4), 546 - 53. http://dx.doi.org/10.1590/ S1516-80342010000400012.

Miller, J. and Schwanenflugel, P. J. (2006). Prosody of syntactically complex sentences in the oral reading of young children. *Journal of educational psychology,* 98(4), 839. 10.1037/0022-0663.98.4.839.

Millán, J. A. (2008). *The reading in Spain: reading for learning.* Madrid: Fundación Germán Sánchez Ruipérez; Federación de Gremios de Editores de España.

Navas, A. L. G. P., Pinto, J. C. B. R. and Dellisa, P. R. R. (2009). Improvements in the knowledge of the reading fluency processing: from word to text. *Revista da Sociedade Brasileira de Fonoaudiologia*, 14(3), 553 - 559. http://dx.doi.org/10.1590/S1516-80342009000400021.

Oliveira, A. M. D., Cardoso, M. H. and Capellini, S. A. (2012). Characterization of reading processes in students with dyslexia and learning disabilities. *Revista da Sociedade Brasileira de Fonoaudiologia*, 201 - 207. http://dx.doi.org/10.1590/S1516-80342012000200017.

Reid, G. (2016). *Dyslexia: A practitioner's handbook*. John Wiley & Sons.

Santos, B. and Capellini, S. A. (2018). *Remediation program with automatized naming and reading – PRONARLE*. Booktoy: Ribeirão Preto.

Silva, R. C. (2017). *Reading comprehension and receptive vocabulary in the elementary school*. Master, Universidade de São Paulo, São Paulo, Brasil.

Silva, C. and Capellini, S. A. (2010). Efficacy of the reading and phonological remediation program in learning disabilities. *Prófono*, 22(2), 131 - 9. http://dx.doi.org/10.1590/S0104-56872010000200011.

Silva, C. D. and Capellini, S. A. (2015). Efficacy of phonological intervention program in students at risk for dyslexia. *Revista CEFAC*, 1827 - 1837. http://dx.doi.org/10.1590/1982-021620151760215.

Silva, C. and Pereira, F. B. (2019). Performance in receptive vocabulary and reading comprehension testes in elementary school students. *Psicologia:Teoria e Prática*, 21(2), 260 - 276.

Solé, I. (1998). *Reading Strategies*. Porto Alegre: Artmed.

Wolf, M. and Denckla, M. B. (2005). *Rapid Automatized naming and rapid alternating stimulus teste*. Pro-ed: Texas.

In: Dyslexia
Editors: Catia Giaconi et al.
ISBN: 978-1-53617-593-6
© 2020 Nova Science Publishers, Inc.

Chapter 6

DYSLEXIA AND CHINESE LANGUAGE: A CASE STUDY

Catia Giaconi[1], Simone Aparecida Capellini[2],
Noemi Del Bianco and Ilaria D'Angelo[1]
[1]Department of Education, Cultural Heritage
and Tourism, University of Macerata (UNIMC),
Macerata, Italy
[2]Investigation Learning Disabilities Laboratory (LIDA),
Department of Speech and Hearing Sciences,
São Paulo State University "Júlio de Mesquita Filho"
(UNESP), Marilia, São Paulo, Brazil

INTRODUCTION

The project that we are going to illustrate in this chapter represents an important case study able to turn into practice how experiences of University inclusion are achievable, through targeted training courses. The experience is part of the *Inclusion 3.0* project from the Italian

University of Macerata, already presented in various publications (Giaconi, Del Bianco 2018a; Giaconi, Del Bianco 2018b); aimed to create new educational opportunities for students with disabilities with Specific Learning Disorder within the University life. In terms of scientific experimentation, the research is part of studies related to Dyslexia and the Chinese Language, specifically, investigating the characteristics of learning the Chinese Language by people with Dyslexia (Cai and Piccioni, 2017) and relative difficulties (Hua, Mcbride-Chang, Sina and Hongyun, 2006; McBride, Ying, and Leo Man-Lit, 2018).

In our study, we wanted to deepen the characteristics related to the learning of the Chinese Language by Italian students with and without Dyslexia.

The survey conducted wanted to propose a course of University teaching of the Chinese Language which, thanks to specific didactic strategies and tools, allowed to favor the learning even of Italian students with Dyslexia.

THE OBSERVATION OF ERRORS LEARNING CHINESE LANGUAGE: A COMPARATIVE STUDY

In this section, we are going to explain the results of the research that investigate the criticalities and the potentialities in learning the Chinese Language for Italian students with and without Dyslexia.

The analyzed material concerns operational notebooks, videos, error observation forms, and analysis of assessment tests. Thanks to this review it was possible to identify the errors committed by Italian students with and without Dyslexia, in learning oral and written the Chinese Language.

Specifically, the following errors were highlighted:

Dyslexia and Chinese Language 73

- Errors in reading Chinese Language characters;
- Errors in reading the "pinyin";
- Errors in writing Chinese Language characters.

Regarding errors in reading Chinese Language characters, both groups (students with and without Dyslexia) have found a slow, but correct way of reading. The most frequent error in both groups was the incorrect intonation, in fact, in the evaluation tests, very often, the structure of Italian phonetics was used. As a result, the incorrect intonation led to the error of the tonal cadence. Respecting tones in the Chinese Language is a fundamental characteristic, since the change of a tone can change the meaning of the word.

In the group, without Dyslexia there were no errors in the omission of characters during the reading, which, instead, were traced in the group with Dyslexia. We also found in the group of people with Dyslexia the error of replacing some characters with others. It has been hypothesized that this error is due to the similarity of the characters. For example, very often the character "吃" was confused with the character "喝", or the character "多少" with the character "什么". This type of error was not found in the control group.

Only in the group with Dyslexia were errors made in the visual confusion of sounds, in fact, several times the character "吃" has been read as "喝".

The most important aspect, that needs to be emphasized, lies in the absence of errors related to character inversions. As expected, this error did not occur in students without Dyslexia, but, mostly, it was not detected in students with Dyslexia. Finally, no errors are recorded about grammatical reading rules, such as errors in the agreement or the recognition of tense, as the Chinese Language presents a simpler grammatical structure.

Table 1, sets out a case study relating to the errors of a Dyslexic student during learning the Chinese Language.

Table 1. Case study illustrating errors in reading

In this table the errors of a case study are presented. In the character reading test there are essentially some intonation and tone exchange errors, but almost all single characters are read correctly. The intonation errors are not proper and verifiable only in subjects with dyslexia. In fact, even in the reading examination of normal readers, the same type of error was found. It is quite common to make a mistake in tone, especially by students who have been studying for the first time. The reading test ended with the examination of the diction of the three sentences. In the first sentence: 她要什么(What do you want?) we observe the replacement of the last character (什么) with (多少). The second sentence: 我们吃什么(What do you eat?) is read correctly. Few errors are made in the intonation. The same goes for the third and final sentence: 我要喝(you want to drink), the characters are read correctly with some intonation errors.

Concerning the reading of "pinyin", that is the alphabetic transcription of Chinese writing, which therefore provides a clue to the correct pronunciation to be respected. Research results showed that "pinyin" reading in both groups was as expected, more fluid than reading characters.

However, in the group of students with Dyslexia, reading appeared hastier and this led to errors more often. Also, concerning the reading of "pinyin", both groups continued to make the mistake related to the wrong intonation, preferring, in fact, the use of the Italian phonetic structure.

Although "pinyin" indicates which tone should be used to read words, the error of tonal cadence remains in both groups. It has, therefore, been hypothesized that this aspect could be connected to the absence of this characteristic in the Italian language. Only in students with Dyslexia remains the error of omitting a syllable when reading a sentence (in the sentence "Tāmen shì laoshī" is omitted "shì") or to omit a syllable within a word (in the word "Tiàowǔ" the second syllable is omitted).

In the group of students with Dyslexia we found the error of replacing syllables with other syllables, which was not present in the group of students without Dyslexia. For example, "Jiǎozi" was read "Xiǎoqī".

Table 2. Case study illustrating pinyin reading errors

The reading test of an alphabetical text, was structured in two parts: in the first part the single words were presented, while, in the second past simple sentences were submitted. The following errors were found in the test performed by the student with dyslexia:

a. Incorrect intonation: many of the words that are spoken are not of tonal correctness. For example, the word: "mǐfàn" (rice) is read correctly, but the syllable "fàn" appears to be produced with the first tone instead of the fourth.

b. Omission of syllables: in the word "tiàowǔ" (dancing) there is an omission of the second syllable. The sound turns out to be "tiau".

c. Errors related to reading rules in oral production: in this case, by way of example, we report several errors taken from the reading of the last three sentences. In the first sentence "Wǒ shì yìdàlì rén" (I'm italian): "shì" is read as is written. The same error is made in the second sentence: "Tāmen shì laoshī" (they are teachers) where the words "shì" and "laoshī" are pronounced literally. The same error is also recorded the last sentence, indeed, the word "shuǐ" (water) is read as it is composed.

d. Replacement of syllables: in the word "zuo fàn" (cooking), the first syllable is read "gh" instead of "z". Another example is recorded in the word "jiǎozi" (ravioli), in which the first syllable is read "gl" instead of "tɕ".

e. Invention of syllables: in the word "xuèshēng" (student) the final syllable is replaced with one of invention of the boy: "ghen".

Moreover, in the group of Dyslexic student's errors were made in the substitution of syllables (error not present in the reading of the characters) and the tendency to visually confuse the sounds in the oral production (the word "Chànggē" was read "Chūnjuǎn").

Finally, in both groups there were errors related to the production rules of the Chinese Language. As explined before, the respect of the tones was the error that created more problems in both groups given the tonal characteristic of the Chinese Language. Table 2, sets out a case study relating to the errors of a Dyslexic student during learning the Chinese Language.

Finally, we are going to analyse the errors in writing an iconic sign of Chinese Language. The first aspect that emerged in the analysis of the writing was slow and stunted writing by the group with Dyslexia. The average writing time of one iconic sign in the control group was 4.6 seconds while in the group of students with Dyslexia the average writing time is almost doubled, up to 8 seconds. From the observation of the writing, it was also possible to understand that in the group of students with Dyslexia there was a non-fluid and irregular section, not present in the writing of non-Dyslexic students. In none of the two groups were errors related to the respect of the proportions registered but instead, there was a difficulty in following an order and a very precise directionality of the traits.

In the Chinese Language, some sounds may seem similar. That aspect created difficulties in the group of Dyslexic students, as in the dictation test some iconic signs having similar sounds have been transcribed in the wrong way. However, these errors did not occur within the subgroup of students without Dyslexia. If Dyslexic students can omit graphemes within words, this is not found in writing Chinese language. Therefore, no errors were found in the omission of lines in either of the two subgroups.

As for the omission of the characters within a bisyllabic word, this error was found in the group of dyslexic students, often, in fact, the first character was transcribed but the second one was omitted.

Basically, this error is not recorded in the control group. Just as in both groups no omissions of traits were recorded in the composition of the characters, it should be noted that no traits were found that were added to the character.

Furthermore, in neither subgroup, no additions of characters were observed in a bisyllabic word or in a sentence.

As it happened in the reading of the characters, it was observed, that in none of the two subgroups were characters inverted, for example, it was never found that "多少" was written "少多" or that 什么 had been written 么什.

As for the errors in the segmentation of the characters, they were not found in either of the two subgroups. It may be assumed that, unlike alphabetic letters, characters are thought of as images that are more difficult to decompose.

In both groups the error of joining the traits was recorded, thus, neglecting the rules of Chinese writing.

On the contrary, there were no errors in the fusion of the characters, which maintained their proportion and sequence. Only in the group of dyslexic student's non-existent spellings were found. The Chinese character was only partially remembered, often in the first part, and then made up in the second one.

Especially in the group of students with dyslexia, there is the difficulty of respecting the order of the traits that describes a character. For example, some rules impose that in a character the external part must first be executed, then the inner part and finally close the "frame". In the evaluation tasks, however, it was seen that students with dyslexia had difficulty following this rule.

Finally, it was found that students with dyslexia did graphia's trait frequent take back and the presence of excessive pressure in doing the graphic traits.

Also in this case, we propose in table 3 a case study as a concrete example.

Table 3. Case study illustrating errors in writing

In order to observe the mistakes made during the writing of a character, the test was structured in the form of a dictation in which the the professor was asked to pronounce the single character and the student was asked to write, in a given time, the correspondent one. The test consisted of eight individual items and three sentences. Finally, the boy was asked to write a character and a sentence of his choice. The creation of a non-existent character occurs several times. First of all, it can be seen with the writing of the character 我(I). In fact, as can be seen from the figure, the boy first writes the corresponding pinyin and subsequently, a character that does not exist. The same mechanism can be found in the transcription of the sentence 我是.. (I'm…) where, in addition to the wrong character, we also find the omission of the 是(to be). In the writing of the character at will, despite the wording transcribed in pinyin is wrong, the student's intention to write 你好(hello) can be identified.

In the first character, there is an omission of a part, while the second is wrong. Overall the character is non-existent (Figure 1).

During the writing of the sentence at will, the entire syntax is omitted and only a hint is made (Figure 2).

Figure 1. Example of creating a non-existent character.

Figure 2. Omission of an entire syntax.

DESIGN OF INCLUSIVE EDUCATIONAL COURSES FOR THE CHINESE LANGUAGE

After analyzing the error mapping, we are going to present the structure of a course of didactics of the Chinese language addressed also to students with dyslexia. The course was organized within the *Inclusion 3.0* project in collaboration with the Confucius Institute of the University of Macerata. A course of 30 hours of lectures and a Summer School at Beijing Normal University in Beijing was designed to facilitate the learning of the Chinese language by university students with dyslexia.

The group of participants was composed of ten university students from the University of Macerata, of these five with a diagnosis of dyslexia.

The lessons were co-taught by two Chinese language teachers and one Chinese mother tongue.

The planning of an inclusive university course was carried out thanks to the collaboration of the chair of Pedagogy and Special Didactics of the University of Macerata.

To make the course accessible to students with dyslexia, specific teaching strategies were adopted. A platform has therefore been prepared as shown below.

The virtual environment made it possible to collect different materials and was prepared according to particular metacognitive indicators.

Specifically, there were anticipation of the lecture materials, videos for pronunciation and tonality, produced by the mother tongue, videos of lesson contents, materials built with visual learning strategies, exercises to reproduce and listen to the words learned (Figure 3).

As for the tools used to write Chinese characters, a special operating notebook was used, whose pages had drawn squares that re-proposed the morphology of the character.

Figure 3. Platform: example of a lesson.

Within each square there were graphic guides who had the role of helping to have a greater visual-spatial awareness during writing.

To facilitate the self-assessment process of the teaching strategies and tools used, specific data sheets were structured.

The student with dyslexia indicated at the end of each lesson the strengths and weaknesses concerning the lesson, the understanding of the topics and the strategies and tools used that were most useful.

In light of these results it can be stated that the Chinese language could be a valid opportunity also for children with dyslexia. The peculiarity of this oriental language lies in its own writing and reading system.

The Chinese language is, in fact, a logographic system where the characters' map meanings thus minimizing the activation of rules for the conversion of graphemes and phonemes. Nevertheless, if we observe the errors of all the participants with dyslexia in the course, the inversion error is never found in both reading and writing. The error indicated above is related to the phonological process and is typical of the dyslexic condition.

Obviously this is a small research that attempts to advance new perspectives in a field that is still little explored. We then tried to study and reconstruct the peculiarities and criticalities present in learning the Chinese language, by children with Italian dyslexia. We believe that the mapping of errors can be a good starting point for those involved in teaching Chinese with Italian students with and without dyslexia. The potential of the platform and of the videos is of considerable inclusive impact, as also demonstrated by our study.

REFERENCES

Aparecida Capellini, S., Franco dos Santos Liporaci, G., Sellin, L., Herrera Cardoso, M., Giaconi, C., and Del Bianco, N. 2018. "Inclusion and New Technology for Students with Learning Disorders and Attention Deficit with Hiperativity Disorder." *Education Sciences and Society* 9(1): 73-80.

Cai J., and Piccioni A. 2017. "Dislessia e apprendimento di lingue tipologicamente distanti - Il caso del cinese". *EL.LE* 6(3): 349-362.

Gayán Guardiola, J. 2001. "The Evolution of Research on Dyslexia." *Anuario de Psicología* 32(1): 3-30.

Giaconi, C., and Capellini, S. 2015. *Conoscere per includere* [*Know to include*]. Milano: FrancoAngeli.

Giaconi, C., Capellini, S., Del Bianco, N., Taddei, A., and D'Angelo, I. 2019. "Study Empowerment for inclusion." *Education Sciences and Society - Open Access Journal* 9(2): 166-183.

Giaconi, C., and Del Bianco, N. Eds. 2018a. *Inclusione 3.0.* [*Inclusion 3.0.*]. Milano: FrancoAngeli.

Giaconi, C., and Del Bianco, N. Eds. 2018b. In *Azione. Prove di inclusione* [In *Action. Inclusion tests*] Milano: FrancoAngeli.

Giaconi, C., Taddei, A., Del Bianco, N., and Capellini, S. 2018. "Inclusive University didactics and technological devices: a case study." *Education Sciences and Society* 9(1): 191-217.

Hua, S., Mcbride-Chang, C., Sina, W., and Hongyun, L. 2006. "Understanding Chinese developmental dyslexia: Morphological awareness as a core cognitive construct." *Journal of Educational Psychology* 98(1): 122-133.

McBride, C., Ying, W., and Leo Man-Lit, C. 2018. "Dyslexia in Chinese." *Current Developmental Disorders Reports* 5(4): 217-225.

In: Dyslexia
Editors: Catia Giaconi et al.
ISBN: 978-1-53617-593-6
© 2020 Nova Science Publishers, Inc.

Chapter 7

CLINICAL SIGNIFICANCE OF PERCEPTUAL-MOTOR PERFORMANCE AND HANDWRITING OF STUDENTS WITH MIXED SUBTYPE DYSLEXIA

Larissa Sellin, Isabela Pires Metzner and Simone Aparecida Capellini
Investigation Learning Disabilities Laboratory (LIDA),
Department of Speech and Hearing Sciences,
São Paulo State University "Júlio de Mesquita Filho" (UNESP),
Marilia, São Paulo, Brazil

INTRODUCTION

According to Reid (2016) dyslexia refers to differences in individual processing, which are characterized by difficulties at the beginning of literacy, affecting the acquisition of reading, writing, and spelling. In addition, failures in cognitive, phonological and/or visual and memory processes, information retrieval, processing speed, time management, coordination, and automation occur.

Developmental dyslexia, according to Galaburda (2003) is presented as a condition that manifests near the age of three, in which the child demonstrates a delay in verbal development. For the author, dyslexia is considered phonological and occurs due to damage to the superior temporal gyrus and temporoparietal regions, while visual dyslexia is associated with parieto-occipital regions.

In the period of literacy there is an overlap of skills for the occurrence of reading and writing learning, involving cognitive, perceptive, linguistic and motor skills that require the use of the sensory-motor and perceptual components of the student, ie, decoding words and the appropriate motor action for the execution of the motor act of writing (Capellini & Souza, 2008).

Students with developmental dyslexia, more specifically students with mixed subtype, present alterations in motor and visuomotor ability. (Getchell et al., 2007; Tsengn et al., 2007; Ferreti, Mazzoti, e Brizzolara; 2008). Some studies indicate that students with interdisciplinary dyslexia dysfunction have difficulties in bimanual coordination, manual dexterity, and fine motor skills, justifying the occurrence of dysgraphia. (Capellini &; Souza, 2008; Chu, 1997; Summer et al., 2008).

Visual processing can lead to decoding errors made by students with dyslexia, which may interfere with access or retrieval of visual word details. (Talcott, 2000) This deficit can cause difficulties in identifying letters that are mirror images of each other, both in writing and at the time of reading. (Fusco, Germano, & Capellini, 2015).

From these manifestations, it is evident that developmental dyslexia is a genetic-neurological condition that presents the variability of cognitive-linguistic behaviors that should be taken into consideration when defining intervention programs, as well as appropriate assessment procedures that meet the manifestations of dyslexia. (Germano, et al., 2014).

Thus, establishing the handwriting profile of students with dyslexia is extremely important for the discussion of subtype, especially at the time of perceptual-motor investigation and writing quality, if there are differences when analyzed together with students with good academic performance, thus enabling the characterization of this population for differential diagnosis as for interventions in the clinical and educational context.

Therefore, this chapter aims to present the clinical significance of perceptual-motor performance and handwriting of students with an interdisciplinary diagnosis of Mixed Dyslexia and students with good academic performance.

METHOD

This study was conducted after approval by the Research Ethics Committee of the Faculty of Philosophy and Sciences of São Paulo State University "Júlio de Mesquita Filho" (UNESP), Marilia, São Paulo, Brazil, under protocol number 3.098.493.

Nine students of both sexes, aged 9 years to 11 years and 11 months of the 4th and 5th grade of an elementary school of municipal public schools, with average socioeconomic level, participated in this study, divided into two groups:

- *Group I (GI):* composed of 9 students with a multidisciplinary diagnosis of mixed subtype developmental dyslexia;
- *Group II (GII):* composed of 9 students from a municipal school with good academic performance, matched according to sex, education and age group with GI.

INCLUSION AND EXCLUSION CRITERIA

The students from GI, with Interdisciplinary Diagnosis of Developmental Dyslexia, were selected from the evaluation carried out by the interdisciplinary team of the Investigation Learning Disabilities Laboratory (LIDA) composed by Speech Therapists, Neuropsychologist and Occupational Therapist (DSM-V, 2014).

Inclusion criteria were the signing of the Free and Informed Consent Form signed by the parents or guardians and did not perform speech, language, education or psychopedagogic intervention. Failure to meet at least one of these criteria described above would automatically exclude the student from the sample of this study.

The GII students of this study were selected in a public school indicated by their teachers for presenting good academic performance in Portuguese Language and Mathematics. From this indication, the students were submitted to the School Performance Test - TDE (Stein, 1994). Only students in the GII of this study were included, who obtained medium to superior performance. The TDE was applied and analyzed by a speech therapist.

Exclusion criteria for GII were the presence of sensory (hearing and/or visual), cognitive or physical deficits, according to aspects described in school records. Excluded from this study were students already submitted to some kind of speech therapy remediation or who did not write with cursive letters.

The sample size of this study was estimated based on the flow of patients diagnosed with developmental dyslexia at LIDA/FCC/UNESP, thus constituting a convenience sample. Exclusion criteria were no co-occurrence with other neuropsychiatric conditions such as attention deficit disorder (ADHD), coordination development disorder (BDD), anxiety, depression, and others.

The absence of co-occurrence in the diagnoses studied in this study reduced the sample but did not decrease the strength of the evidence of the evaluation findings, since the measures used in the procedures are obtained by score, thus allowing a descriptive analysis of the data by means of obtaining the mean and standard deviation values and statistical treatment with non-parametric teste.

The GI students were evaluated in classrooms of the Specialized Rehabilitation Center - CER/FFC/UNESP - Marília-SP, in a period contrary to the school period and GII students were evaluated in the schools of origin in the school period. The application of the TDE writing and math tests to the GII was applied as a group in a single session.

All students in this study were submitted the following procedures.

Visual Perception Development Test III - DTVP III (Hammill, Pearson, & Voress, 2014)

This test consists of a battery of five subtests that measure different visual-motor and visual-perceptual skills. It can be applied for four purposes, namely: (a) identifying children with visual impairment or visual perception problems, (b) determining the severity of these problems, (c) verifying the effectiveness of intervention programs designed to correct the problems, and (d) to serve as a measurement tool in research and research. All subtests measure a type of visual reception ability and can be considered as reduced motricity subtests (bottom figure, visual closure, and shape constancy), overall visual perception (copy, eye-hand coordination, bottom figure, visual closure), and shape constancy), visuomotor integration (copying and eye-hand coordination).

The subtests that make up the DTVP-III and were applied to the population of this study:

- *Visual-motor coordination (CVM):* Students were asked to accurately draw a straight line and/or curve, in accordance with the visual limits.
- *Copy (C):* A simple figure was presented to the student and required to draw it on a piece of paper. The figure is used as a template for copying/drawing;
- *Figure - Background (FF):* The students were presented with some pictures (stimuli) and required to find as many pictures as they can on a page, which will be hidden in a complex background;
- *Visual Closure (CV):* The student was presented with a picture/stimulus and required to select exactly that stimulus from a series of other pictures that were incompletely drawn. In order to complete and finish the test, children will have to mentally provide the missing parts of the pictures in the series;
- *The constancy of form (FC):* The student was presented with a target figure (stimulus) and required to find it within a series of figures. The target figure will have a different size, position and/or hue and can be hidden within a distinct image.

The DTVP-III score is divided into standard score, which is obtained from the gross score and its conversion using tables, and the composite score, obtained by summing the standard scores and converting them into a classification quotient relative to the general visual perception, reduced motricity perception and visuomotor integration. The subtests were applied in the following order: (1) Visuomotor Coordination, (2) Copy, (3) Figure - Bottom, (4) Visual Closure, (5) Shape Constancy. All subtests were applied individually and could not be in a group in a distraction-free, well-ventilated, well-lit, quiet and comfortable environment.

Dysgraphia Scale

The analysis of writing was performed through the application of the Dysgraphia Scale (Lorenzini, 1993), composed of 10 evaluation items, namely: Floating Lines; Ascending/Descending Lines; Irregular Space between Words; Retouched letters; Angulation Bends of the Arcades of the M, N, U, V; Junction points; Collisions and adhesions; Sudden movements; Irregularity of Dimensions and More Forms. Students were asked to copy the following note:

> "My dear friend:
> I'm very glad to see you on Thursday.
> If the weather is good, we will go for a walk.
> Affectionately."

The scoring criterion used to analyze the writing performance of the students in this study is the one proposed by Lorenzini (1993), and the overall grade for each writing ranged from zero to seventeen points, and then all subjects with a grade equal to or greater than one were considered dysgraphic greater than eight and a half points - equivalent to 50% of the total grade.

The analysis of the results was performed using the JT (Del Prette & Del Prette, 2008) Method which provides a comparative analysis between scores in order to decide if the differences between them represent reliable changes and if they are clinically relevant.

RESULTS

Graph 1 shows the performance in the sub-tests of visual-motor coordination, copy, background-figure, visual closure and shape constancy of students with mixed dyslexia compared with students with good academic performance.

Graph 1. Index of positive and negative reliable change in students with mixed dyslexia and good academic performance of DTVP III.

Table 1. Characterization of the writing analysis of students with mixed dyslexia using the dysgraphia scale

People	LF	LAD	EI	LR	CAA	PJ	CA	MB	ID	MF	Total	Writing Classification
1	2	0,5	0,5	1	0	1	1,5	1	0	1	8,5	Dysgraphic
2	1	1	1	1	0	1	3	2	2	1	13	Dysgraphic
3	1	1	0,5	0	0	1	3	2	2	1	11,5	Dysgraphic
4	1	1	1	1	0	1	3	0	1	1	10	Dysgraphic
5	2	1	1	1	0	0	1,5	2	2	1	11,5	Dysgraphic
6	1	0,5	1	1	0	1	1,5	1	1	0,5	8,5	Dysgraphic
7	1	1	1	2	0	0	1,5	2	2	1	11,5	Dysgraphic
8	1	0,5	1	1	0	1	1,5	1	1	0,5	8,5	Dysgraphic
9	2	0,5	1	2	0	2	1	2	2	1	12,5	Dysgraphic

Caption: LF: Floating Lines; LAD: Ascending and descending lines; EI: Irregular space between words; LR: Retouched letters; CAA: Curvatures and angulations of the arcades of M, N, U, V; PJ: junction points; CA: Collisions and adhesions; MB: sudden movements; ID: Dimension irregularity; MF: Bad forms.

This Graph 1 shows the number of comparisons in which the reliable change index was negative (in red) and when the reliable change index was positive (in blue), that is, students with mixed dyslexia performed poorly on the copy subtests, background figure, visual closure and shape constancy in relation to students with good academic performance. In the visual-motor coordination subtest, there was no discrepancy regarding the performance of students with mixed dyslexia and students with good academic performance.

The Table 1 presents the scores achieved by dyslexic students on the dysgraphia scale (Lorenzini, 1993). From the table above, it is possible to observe that all students with mixed dyslexia scored sufficiently to be considered dysgraphic (8.5).

DISCUSSION

Based on the data obtained, it was observed that all students with mixed dyslexia (GI) presented dysgraphic writing quality in relation to the group with good academic performance (GII) referring to the Dysgraphia Scale procedure (Lorenzini, 1993). In the DTVP - III subtests, it was possible to observe from the graph above that the students with Mixed Dyslexia presented a lower performance in the copy, figure - bottom, visual closure and shape constancy subtests compared to the students with good academic performance.

According to the literature, the presence of dysgraphia in students with dyslexia suggests the existence of alterations in letter tracing in tasks involving copying, and manual dexterity. (Fawcett & Nicolson, 2011; Capellini & Souza, 2008). Studies have shown that students with dyslexia present changes in motor skills, involving difficulty in bimanual coordination, manual dexterity, and fine motor skills, justifying the occurrence of dysgraphia. (Getchell; et al., 2007; Jefferies, Sage, & Ralph, 2007; Crawford & Dewey, 2008).

The study by Capellini, Coppede & Valle (2010) states that fine, sensory and perceptive motor alterations are responsible for the dysgraphic picture of students with dyslexia, and there is a correlation between the absence of dysgraphia in tests of fine motor, sensory and perceptive in the group of students with good academic performance, which corroborates the study of this chapter, in which all students with Mixed Dyslexia presented dysgraphic writing quality, while the group of students with good academic performance did not present dysgraphia.

Concerning the perceptual-motor function, according to Brow & Rodger (2008), there is a combination of the visuomotor, motor, cognitive, perceptual skills (eye-hand coordination) position in space, spatial relationship, background, and constancy of form. Thus, students with dyslexia are prone to presenting manifestations of visual perceptual changes due to dysfunctions in the brain areas responsible for visuospatial perception, which is responsible at the time of writing. (Wang & Su, 2009; Fusco, Okuda, & Capellini, 2011).

According to the study by Germano, Pinheiro, Okuda, and Capellini (2011), students with Attention Deficit Hyperactivity Disorder (ADHD) showed poorer performance in visuomotor perception skills when compared to students with good academic performance, being they characterized by impaired perception of reduced motor skills, involving tasks of position in space, background figure, visual closure and shape constancy, in addition to changes in visual-motor integration, which corroborates this study in the variables copy, background figure, closure. There was a statistically significant difference between the group of students with mixed dyslexia and the group of students with good academic performance, in which the group with dyslexia.

Thus, it is considered that the difficulty in performing the visual-motor perception and visual perception skills in these students compromises the performance of handwriting, and dysgraphia may occur as described in the literature. (Toniolo et al., 2009; Racine, Majnemer, Shevell & 2008).

CONCLUSION

The results show that the students with Mixed Dyslexia (GI) had a poor performance in the copy, background figure, visual closure, and shape constancy in the DTVP - III compared to the students with good academic performance.

Regarding the analysis of writing, GI presented a higher frequency of students with dysgraphia, showing fine motor sensory and perceptive alterations, which are directly responsible for the dysgraphic picture of this group. Regarding the absence of dysgraphia in the GII, it is evident that students without dyslexia develop the practice of fine and global motor skills.

REFERENCES

American Psychiatric Association. (2014). *DSM-V: Manual diagnóstico e estatístico de Transtornos Mentais* [*Diagnostic and Statistical Manual of Mental Disorders*].

Chu, S. (1997). Occupational therapy for children with handwriting difficulties: A framework for evaluation and treatment. *British Journal of Occupational Therapy, 60*(12), 514-520. Available in: 10.1177/030802269706001202.

Del Prette, Z. A. P., Del Prette, Clinical Significance and Reliable Change in Evaluating Psychological Interventions. *Psicologia: teoria e pesquisa*. 2008; 24(4): 497-505. Available in: 10.1590/S0102377220080000400013.

Ferretti, G., Mazzotti, S., & Brizzolara, D. (2008). Visual scanning and reading ability in normal and dyslexic children. *Behavioural Neurology, 19*(1-2), 87-92. Available in: 10.1155/2008/564561.

Fusco, N., Germano, G. D., & Capellini, S. A. (2015, April). Efficacy of a perceptual and visual-motor skill intervention program for students with dyslexia. In *CoDAS* (Vol. 27, No. 2, pp. 128-134). Sociedade Brasileira de Fonoaudiologia. Available in: 10.1590/2317-1782/20152014013.

Galaburda, A. M., & Cestnick, L. (2003). Dislexia del desarrollo. [Developmental dyslexia] *Revista de neurología*, *36*(1), 3-9. Available in: 10.33588/rn.36S1.2003068.

Germano, G. D., Reilhac, C., Capellini, S. A., & Valdois, S. (2014). The phonological and visual basis of developmental dyslexia in Brazilian Portuguese reading children. *Frontiers in psychology*, *5*, 1169. Available in: 10.3389/fpsyg.2014.01169.

Getchell, N., Pabreja, P., Neeld, K., & Carrio, V. (2007). Comparing children with and without dyslexia on the movement assessment battery for children and the test of gross motor development. *Perceptual and motor skills*, *105*(1), 207-214. Available in: 10.2466/PMS.105.5.207-214.

Reid, G. (2016). Dyslexia: A practitioner's handbook. John Wiley & Sons. Summers, J., Larkin, D., & Dewey, D. (2008). Activities of daily living in children with developmental coordination disorder: dressing, personal hygiene, and eating skills. *Human movement science*, *27*(2), 215-229. Available in: 10.1016/j.humov.2008.02.002.

Talcott, J. B., Hansen, P. C., Assoku, E. L., & Stein, J. F. (2000). Visual motion sensitivity in dyslexia: evidence for temporal and energy integration deficits. *Neuropsychologia*, *38*(7), 935-943. Available in: 10.1016/s0028-3932(00)00020-8.

Trevisan, J. G., Coppede, A. C., & Capellini, S. A. (2008). Fine motor, sensory and perceptive function of students with attention deficit disorder with hyperactivity. *Temas desenvolv*, *16*(94), 183-187. Available in: 10.1590/S2179-64912011000400010.

Tseng, M. H., & Chow, S. M. (2000). Perceptual-motor function of school-age children with slow handwriting speed. *American Journal of Occupational Therapy*, *54*(1), 83-88. Available in: 10.5014/ajot.54.1.83.

In: Dyslexia ISBN: 978-1-53617-593-6
Editors: Catia Giaconi et al. © 2020 Nova Science Publishers, Inc.

Chapter 8

CHARACTERIZATION OF FINE MOTOR FUNCTION IN STUDENTS WITH DEVELOPMENTAL DYSLEXIA

Giseli Donadon Germano,
Raíssa Angleni Machado Pereira
and Simone Aparecida Capellini
Investigation Learning Disabilities Laboratory (LIDA),
Department of Speech and Hearing Sciences,
São Paulo State University "Júlio de Mesquita Filho"
(UNESP), Marilia, São Paulo, Brazil

INTRODUCTION

Studies describe that students with dyslexia may manifest difficulties in acquiring and controlling fine motor skills, which interfere with the quality of handwriting (Tseng and Chow 2000). Among the justifications for these alterations, Smits-Engelsman,

Niemeijer and van Galen (2001) report that the movement difficulties of students with dyslexia reflect a reduced ability to automate motor skills.

This difficulty would be related to the deficit in working memory and/or selective attention that would not be well integrated (or fragmented) in the learning process.

Consequently, the information for performing a task is not sufficiently memorized, not generating motor program memories. Thus, when asked to perform a task, the student has the impression that he is performing a totally "new" task, while other information still needs to be processed. Because of this, the student has more need for feedback during the execution of the movement and cannot anticipate and plan future strategies (Smits-Engelsman, Wilson, Westenberg and Duysens 2003).

Another aspect worth mentioning refers to the use of working memory.

The impairment in working memory has been related as a consistent finding and observed in students with dyslexia. The nature of the link between impaired verbal working memory and dyslexia has been referred to as complicated by the fact that mechanisms that allow information to be retained for a given time depend on the access of this representation at long-term memory.

These long-term memory representations correspond to representations stored in the language system (Majerus and Cowan 2016).

Thus, to produce skilled movement, sequentially coordinated muscle activation is required. It is generally assumed that such movements are controlled by memorized motor programs and contain the appropriate muscle commands for the next movement (Gordon, Forssberg, Johansson and Westling 1991).

Among the motor alterations, there is the fine motor function, which requires a greater degree of integration and proper functioning of the central nervous system, being characterized as the ability to control a set of movement activities of certain body segments, with employment minimum strength in order to achieve a goal, efficiently and precisely to the task (Silveira, Gobbi, Caetano, Rossi and Candido 2005; Okuda et al. 2011). Thus, fine motor skills (or precision) refer to the use of small hand muscles for hand manipulation, proper use of the tool, and mature patterns of grasping and grasping (Bruininks and Bruininks 2005).

Thus, fine motor function involves the coordination of visual-motor skills coordination with motor planning, cognitive planning with perceptual skills, and visual-motor integration. Visual-motor integration, described as the ability to coordinate visual information with motor programming, is directly related to school learning processes, being important in students' academic life, during the production of handwriting, in activities such as copying and text production (Brown and Rodger 2008).

Thus, changes in some of these skills may cause academic impairment.

In this way, this study hypothesizes that students with dyslexia might experience difficulties in fine motor function due to failures in precision or fine motor integration. So, the aim of this study was to characterize and compare fine motor function in students with dyslexia with good academic performance.

METHOD

This study was conducted after approval by the Research Ethics Committee of the Faculty of Philosophy and Sciences of São Paulo State University "Júlio de Mesquita Filho" (UNESP), Marilia, São Paulo, Brazil, under the number 2.017.705.

A total of 20 students participated of this study, of both sexes, with age from 8 years to 11 years and 11 months of age, from 3rd to 5th grade level of Elementary School I, who attend municipal public education. The students will be divided into groups:

Group I (GI): composed with 10 students with interdisciplinary diagnosis of dyslexia.

Group II (GII): composed with 10 students with good academic performance, paired with GI in relation to sex and chronological age.

Students from GI groups were selected based on the evaluation performed by the interdisciplinary team, composed by Speech Language Therapists, Neuropsychologists and Occupational Therapists, based on the criteria described in the Diagnostic and statistical manual of mental disorders - DSM-V (American Psychiatric Association, APA 2013).

The students of GII were considered with good academic performance those with satisfactory performance in two consecutive assessment of Portuguese Language and Mathematics, and performance higher than or equal to the average (5.0). In addition, students with classification of performance from "medium" to "superior" in the reading, writing and arithmetic tests in the School Performance Test (Stein 1994).

The students underwent Bruininks-Oseretsky Motor Assessment Test of Motor Proficiency 2 - BOT-2 (Bruininks and Bruininks 2005). The procedure consists of a set of tests, which evaluate motor areas. This study used the fine motor evaluation part, composed of the Fine Motor Precision and Fine Motor Integration, which together form the composite score Fine Manual Control subtest. The subtests measure the motor skills involved in writing and drawing, tasks that require precise control of finger and hand movements.

The students were evaluated individually, lasting between 20 and 40 minutes, in a quiet room. All conversions were performed from reference tables proposed by the protocol for each chronological age and sex. The students were classified in relation to the composite scores, being much below average (score 0), below average (1), average (2), above average (3), much above average (4).

RESULTS

The results were statistically analyzed using the following Statistical Package for the Social Sciences software (SPSS, version 20) and Excel Office 2010. The Mann-Whitney Test was performed (in order to verify a possible difference between the groups studied) and the Chi-square test to verify frequencies regarding the protocol classification. It was considered a significance level of p-values considered statistically significant before the adopted significance level (0.05), indicated by an asterisk (*).

Table 1 shows the mean, standard deviation (SD), and p value for the latency variable when comparing groups GI and GII for Fine Motor Precision (FMP), Fine Motor Integration (FMI), and Fine Manual Control (FMC) and classification (CL).

It can be observed in Table 1 that there was significant difference among students of GI and GII for fine motor precision and classification, and GI performance was lower than GII. There was also a significant difference between the groups for Fine Manual Control and its classification, with lower GI performance than GII.

Table 1. Mean distribution, standard deviation (SD), and p value in the comparison between GI and GII

	GI		GII		
	Mean	SD	Mean	SD	P value
FMP	9.9	5.238	16.8	4.638	0.008*
CL_FMP	1.3	0.823	2.3	0.675	0.011*
FMI	11.1	3.281	13	3.972	0.253
CL_FMI	1.5	0.527	1.8	0.632	0.282
FMC	40.1	10.126	50	7.394	0.023*
CF_FMC	1.4	0.843	2.2	0.422	0.015*

Caption: FMP: Fine Motor Precision; IMF: Fine Motor Integration; FMC: Fine Manual Control; CL: classification. Mann-Whitney Test (* $p < 0.05$).

Since the Classification of Fine Manual Control is based on the sum of Fine Motor Precision and Fine Motor Integration (not significant), this findings may suggest that the difficulties of students with dyslexia were caused by failures in Fine Motor Precision, which verifies the precise control of finger and hand movements, affecting their performance in coloring shapes, maze lines, connecting dots, folding paper and scissors cutting circles.

Table 2. Classification distribution (CL) for Fine Motor Precision (FMP), Fine Motor Integration (IMF) and Fine Manual Control (FMC) of GI and GII students

	Classification	GI N Observed (%)	GII N Observed (%)
CL_FMP	Very below average	1 (10%)	0 (0%)
	below average	6 (60%)	1 (10%)
	average	2 (20%)	5 (50%)
	Above average	1 (10%)	4 (40%)
	Total	10 (100%)	10 (100%)
	P value	0,187	
CL_FMI	Very below average	0 (0%)	0 (0%)
	below average	5 (50%)	3 (30%)
	average	5 (50%)	6 (60%)
	Above average	0 (0%)	1 (10%)
	Total	10 (100%)	10 (100%)
	P value	0,019*	
CL_FMC	Very below average	1 (10%)	0 (0%)
	below average	5 (50%)	0 (0%)
	average	3 (30%)	8 (80%)
	Above average	1 (10%)	2 (20%)
	Total	10 (100%)	10 (100%)
	P value	0,011*	

Chi-square test (* $p < 0.05$).

Table 2 presents the classification of frequency distribution for the Fine Motor Precision (FMP), Fine Motor Integration (FMI) and Fine Manual Control (FMC) variables, from the Chi-Square test.

Table 2 shows that the majority of GI students (90%) performed below average for Fine Motor Precision while for GII, 90% presented average or above average performance. However, there was no significant difference. No students performed Very above average.

Regarding the classification of Fine Motor Integration (IMF) and Fine Manual Control (FMC), there was a significant difference between the groups. For IMF, 50% of students with dyslexia performed on average, while 70% of students with good academic performance performed on average and above average. Regarding the FMC, 60% of students with dyslexia performed below average, while 100% of students with good academic performance performed on average and above average.

These findings suggest that students with dyslexia have difficulties with Fine Motor Integration (FMI), even though they are not significant in relation to the BOT-2 classification. The findings also indicate difficulties in relation to Fine Manual Control (FMC), which corresponds to the sum of the FMP and FMI scores. Thus, we can infer that the difficulties of dyslexic students in FMC would be related to the FMP component, as shown in Table 1.

DISCUSSION

The findings of this study indicated that students with dyslexia had difficulties regarding fine motor precision skills and their classification and for Fine Manual Control and their classification. Since the Classification of Fine Manual Control is based on the sum of Fine Motor Precision and Fine Motor Integration (not significant), we may suggest that the difficulties of students with dyslexia were caused by failures in Fine Motor Precision, which verifies the precise control of finger and hand movements, such as coloring shapes, maze lines, connecting dots, folding paper and scissors cutting circles.

In the international literature (Loh and Piek 2011; Rosemblum 2008) and in the national literature (Germano, Giaconi and Capellini 2016), studies report that students with dyslexia present fine and global motor coordination problems as well as indicate a relationship between the alterations of visuomotor perception and reading and handwriting performance of these students.

Thus, fine motor skills (or dexterity) refer to the use of small hand muscles for hand manipulation, proper use of the tool and mature grasping and grasping patterns. Hand manipulation skills include translation (linear movement of an object from palm to fingers or fingers to palm), simple rotation (movement of an object less than 180 degrees around an axis using isolated finger and thumb movements), complex rotation movement of an object more than 180 degrees around an axis using isolated finger and thumb movements) and change (alternating finger and thumb pad movements). Motor separation on both sides of the hand is an important component of developing fine motor skills, which enables the skilled fingers on the radial side of the hand (thumb, index, and middle finger) to perform small, coordinated, skillful movements, and the powerful ulnar portion of the hand (ring and toes) to provide additional muscle strength during prolonged seizure of the items (Bruininks and Bruininks 2005).

In a broad context, the precision of movement depends on spatial perception, which is based on various senses, such as sight, touch, hearing, balance, and proprioceptive information. Among them, the authors highlight that there is an important relationship between movement coordination and visual feedback, allowing corrections and changes in the direction of the stroke used to handwriting activies (Tous-Ral, Muiños, Liutsko and Forero 2012).

In addition, the findings of this study corroborate studies that suggest a possible co-occurrence of motor, cognitive and social skills.

The authors argue for the presence of neurobiological evidence that supports specific relationships between cognitive and motor development. Motor development, especially the development of fine motor skills, requires neural networks and pathways that substantially overlap those underlying cognitive development (Floyer-Lea and Matthews 2004; Pangelinan et al. 2011; Kim, Carlson, Curby and Winsler 2016).

There are several conjectures as to why motor and language problems co-occur. For one thing, they can be different comorbid problems with a common genetic background. Researchers have widely accepted that, at least in part, dyslexia have a genetic basis (Pennington 1999; Grigorenko 2001). On the other hand, it may be that language and motor problems share a common underlying neurocognitive mechanism. One possible explanation may be related to temporal processing (e.g., time, precision and serial ordering), altered in students with dyslexia.

Thus, also collaborating with Smits-Engelsman et al. (2003), the deficit of students with dyslexia would be related to the programming of fast and precise movements. This indicates that students rely more on feedback, such as visual (indirect component of the Fine Motor Integration – IMF), during the execution of the movement. The authors also point out that such difficulty would be related to the deficit in working memory and/or selective attention that would not be well integrated (or fragmented) in the learning process.

Conclusion

We conclude that students with dyslexia had difficulties in fine motor skills and their classification and for Fine Manual Control and their classification, suggesting integration failures between movement coordination and visual feedback. The findings allow inferring that students with dyslexia fail to retain information to perform a task not sufficiently memorized, not generating memories of motor programs.

These findings have important clinical and educational implications, bringing to the discussion the need for systematic and explicit teaching of fine motor function activities for the school population. In addition, the findings show that there is a need for further investigation of the fine motor function profile in students with dyslexia, which may contribute to improved diagnosis and multidisciplinary therapeutic planning.

Finally, as a limitation of this study, we highlight the small number of subjects per group, suggesting the need for further studies with this population.

REFERENCES

American Psychiatric Association. (2013). *Diagnostic and statistical manual of mental disorders* (DSM-5®). American Psychiatric Pub.

Brown, T. and Rodger, S. (2008). Validity of the developmental test of visual-motor integration supplemental developmental test of visual perception. *Perceptual and motor skills,* 106(3), 659 - 678. Doi: 10.2466/pms.106.3.659-678.

Bruininks, R. H. and Bruininks, B. D. (2005). *BOT2: Bruininks-oseretsky Test of Motor Proficiency*. Pearson.

Floyer-Lea, A. and Matthews, P. M. (2004). Changing brain networks for visuomotor control with increased movement automaticity. *Journal of Neurophysiology,* 92(4), 2405 - 2412. Doi: 10.1152/jn.01092.2003.

Germano, G. D., Giaconi, C. and Capellini, S. A. (2016). Characterization of brazilians students with dyslexia in Handwriting Proficiency Screening Questionnaire and Handwriting Scale.

Psychology Research, 6(10), 590 - 7. Doi: doi:10.17265/2159-5542/2016.10.004.

Gordon, A. M., Forssberg, H., Johansson, R. S. and Westling, G. (1991). Visual size cues in the programming of manipulative forces during precision grip. *Experimental brain research*, 83(3), 477 - 482. Doi: 10.1007/BF00229824.

Grigorenko, E. L. (2001). Developmental dyslexia: An update on genes, brains, and environments. *The Journal of Child Psychology and Psychiatry and Allied Disciplines,* 42(1), 91 - 125. Doi: 10.1017/S0021963001006564.

Kim, H., Carlson, A. G., Curby, T. W. and Winsler, A. (2016). Relations among motor, social, and cognitive skills in pre-kindergarten children with developmental disabilities. *Research in developmental disabilities*, 53, 43 - 60. Doi: 10.1016/j.ridd.2016.01.016.

Loh, P. R., Piek, J. P. and Barrett, N. C. (2011). Comorbid ADHD and DCD: Examining cognitive functions using the WISC-IV. *Research in developmental disabilities,* 32(4), 1260 - 1269. Doi: 10.1016/j.ridd.2011.02.008.

Majerus, S. and Cowan, N. (2016). The nature of verbal short-term impairment in dyslexia: The importance of serial order. *Frontiers in Psychology*, 7, 1522. Doi: 10.3389/fpsyg.2016.01522.

Okuda, P. M. M., Pinheiro, F. H., Germano, G. D., Padula, N. A. D. M. R., Lourencetti, M. D., Santos, L. C. A. D. and Capellini, S. A. (2011). Fine motor, sensory and perceptive function of students with attention deficit disorder with hyperactivity. *Jornal da Sociedade Brasileira de Fonoaudiologia*, 23(4), 351 - 357. Doi: 10.1590/S2179-64912011000400010.

Pangelinan, M. M., Zhang, G., VanMeter, J. W., Clark, J. E., Hatfield, B. D. and Haufler, A. J. (2011). Beyond age and gender: relationships between cortical and subcortical brain volume and cognitive-motor abilities in school-age children. *Neuroimage*, 54(4), 3093 - 3100. Doi: 10.1016/j.neuroimage.2010.11.021.

Pennington, B. F. (1999). Toward an integrated understanding of dyslexia: Genetic, neurological, and cognitive mechanisms. *Development and Psychopathology*, 11(3), 629 - 654. Doi: 10.1017/ S0954579499002242.

Rosenblum, S. (2008). Development, reliability, and validity of the Handwriting Proficiency Screening Questionnaire (HPSQ). *American Journal of Occupational Therapy*, 62(3), 298 - 307.

Silveira, C. R. A., Gobbi, L. T. B., Caetano, M. J. D., Rossi, A. C. S. and Candido, R. P. (2005). Avaliação motora de pré-escolares: relações entre idade motora e idade cronológica [Motor assessment of preschoolers: relationships between motor age and chronological age]. *Lecturas: Educación Física y Deportes*, 83, 1 - 5, 2005.

Smits-Engelsman, B. C., Niemeijer, A. S. and van Galen, G. P. (2001). Fine motor deficiencies in children diagnosed as DCD based on poor grapho-motor ability. *Human movement science*, 20(1 - 2), 161 - 182. Doi: 10.1016/S0167-9457(01)00033-1.

Smits-Engelsman, B. C. M., Wilson, P. H., Westenberg, Y. and Duysens, J. (2003). Fine motor deficiencies in children with developmental coordination disorder and learning disabilities: An underlying open-loop control deficit. *Human movement science*, 22(4 - 5), 495 - 513. Doi: 10.1016/j.humov.2003.09.006.

Stein, L. M. (1994). *TDE: teste de desempenho escolar: manual para aplicação e interpretação*. São Paulo: Casa do Psicólogo, 1 - 17.

Tous-Ral, J. M., Muiños, R., Liutsko, L. and Forero, C. G. (2012). Effects of sensory information, movement direction, and hand use on fine motor precision. *Perceptual and Motor Skills*, 115(1), 261 - 272. Doi: 10.2466/25.22.24.PMS.115.4.261-272.

Tseng, M. H. and Chow, S. M. (2000). Perceptual-motor function of school-age children with slow handwriting speed. *American Journal of Occupational Therapy*, 54(1), 83 - 88. Doi: 10.5014/ ajot.54.1.83.

Viholainen, H., Ahonen, T., Cantell, M., Lyytinen, P. and Lyytinen, H. (2002). Development of early motor skills and language in children at risk for familial dyslexia. *Developmental Medicine and Child Neurology,* 44(11), 761 - 769. Doi: 10.1017/S0012162201002894.

In: Dyslexia
Editors: Catia Giaconi et al.
ISBN: 978-1-53617-593-6
© 2020 Nova Science Publishers, Inc.

Chapter 9

VISUAL PERCEPTION STUDIES IN THE ITALIAN LANGUAGE

Ilaria Dángelo[1], Noemi Del Bianco[1],
Simone Aparecida Capellini[2] and Catia Giaconi[1]

[1]Dipartimento di Scienze della Formazione, dei Beni Culturali e del Turismo, Università degli Studi di Macerata (UNIMC), Macerata, Italy
[2]Investigation Learning Disabilities Laboratory (LIDA), Department of Speech and Hearing Sciences, São Paulo State University "Júlio de Mesquita Filho" (UNESP), Marilia, São Paulo, Brazi

INTRODUCTION

When we ask ourselves about the difficulties associated with school learning, attention is often paid to verbal cognitive processes and the role they play in the acquisition of reading, writing, and calculation. However, in order to acquire these skills, efficient non-verbal functions are also needed, such as visual-spatial skills (Fastame, Antonini, 2011). In fact, many components of spatiality, orientation, eye-manual coordination and visual discrimination of the elements are involved in the learning of reading, writing and computational operations (Capellini, Giaconi, 2015).

The pioneering studies of Baddeley and Hitch (1974) have highlighted the central role played by Working Memory (WM), and in particular by the Visual-Space Working Memory (VSWM), in different complex cognitive tasks such as reasoning, understanding, and learning (Baddeley, 1986). The WM is involved in maintaining and connecting information during the execution of tasks such as the non-verbal reasoning (Fatame, Antolini 2011; Baddeley 1986), in the learning of new knowledge, in solving problems and in "formulating and establishing relationships for the achievement of specific objectives" (Mammarella et al., 2008, p. 16).

The WM is, therefore, implicated in the processes of focusing attention and in decision making during the simultaneous performance of other complex activities, through the selection of relevant information for the execution of the task (Zaccaria, 2008). The VSWM, part of the larger mnestic system of the WM, is specifically delegated to temporarily preserve visual and spatial information in order to make it available for the execution of imaginative tasks (Mammarella, 2008). Its role is central in various school disciplines in which the manipulation of mental images, the comparison between visual stimuli and their active processing is required (Mammarella, 2008; Fastame, Antonini, 2011). Given the centrality of these processes and given the studies in Brazil, which are presented in this book, we are going to present the state of the art in the Italian context and, subsequently, a research perspective in Italian school contexts.

STUDIES AND PROCEDURES IN THE ITALIAN CONTEXT

Recognizing the importance of an accurate analysis of visual-spatial skills in order to highlight specific difficulties and consequently identify alternative educational activities, various assessment tools have been developed. Among those validated in the Italian context and most used in the clinical setting, we recall *The Rey Complex Figure* (RCF) (1967), a test that consists of the graphic reproduction of a complex two-dimensional figure and its recall to memory after an interval of three minutes. The test is considered useful for the evaluation of the development of visual-spatial functions, visual-graphic memory and some aspects of planning and executive functions (Caffarra et al., 2001).

Another test is *Visual-Motor Integration* (VMI; Beery and Buktenica, 2000) that allows appreciating a person's abilities to integrate visual and motor skills. The test consists of presenting progressively more complex geometric images that will have to be copied. There are different skills evaluated by VMI such as "the perception, mental representation, motor planning, and graphic reproduction" (Mammarella et al., 2008, p. 18). An additional test used in clinical practice is the *Test of visual perception and visual-motor integration* (TPV; Hammill et al., 1994) which constitutes the revision of the *Developmental Test of Visual Perception* by Frostig, Lefever, and Whittlesey (1974).

The test assesses general visual perception and visual-motor integration through eight subtests that foresee different degrees of motor involvement. Other tests can be obtained from intelligence tests, such as the *Spatial Relations Test* of the *PMA* (Thurstone and Thurstone, 1985) or, from the *TEMA* battery (Reynolds and Bigler, 1995), the subtest Memory of faces; Memory of objects; Abstract visual memory; Visual sequential memory; Spatial location memory.

The tests mentioned above identify a common critical issue. As pointed out by Mammarella et al., (2008), in the execution of the various tests, numerous are the skills employed. Although all related to the field of visual-spatial abilities, the execution of tasks in which perceptual, praxis, visual memory, graphic reproduction, etc. are involved at the same time does not allow us to identify and "isolate the individual processes" (Ivi, p. 13). This makes difficult to understand the specific difficulties that the test performer runs into and, therefore, to arrive at the adoption of useful solutions. Moreover, some tests create confusion between what is the presentation format of a stimulus and the process or strategy used by a participant to face a task (Mammarella, 2008, p. 31).

In the desire to overcome these difficulties, batteries were developed for the evaluation of visual-spatial memory that adopts as a theoretical model the *Continua* model of Cornoldi and Vecchi (2003), proposing tests based on a differentiation of the components of Working Memory.

There have been several theoretical conceptualizations of the WM model (Baddeley and Hitch 1974; Baddeley, 1986; Loggie, 1995) which articulate its structure into a central control component, the Central Executive, and in a series of subsidiary, functionally independent systems of which the best known are the Articulatory Loop and the Visual-Spatial Scratchpad (Fastame, Antonini, 2011, p. 17-18). More recently, Cornoldi and Vecchi (2003) have proposed a new articulation of the model, introducing a representation of the structures forming the WM system according to two continuous dimensions (the *horizontal continuum* and the *vertical continuums*). This has led to the distinction in WM, both in verbal and visuospatial terms, between passive and active tasks and between simultaneous and contemporary processes. The passive task differs from the active one due to the lower cognitive expenditure. In fact, it just requires to keep the information available that, instead, must be developed and transformed into the active task (Mammarella et al., 2008).

Sequential processes are activated in the presentation of a sequence of stimuli whose position must be maintained or processed, while the contemporary processes are activated in the simultaneous presentation of more information. This determines a fundamental difference in the structuring of tests for the evaluation of the VSWM between tasks presented according to a visual format, in which the stimuli differ in shape or texture, a spatial-sequential tasks, in which the order of presentation plays a crucial role, and a spatial-simultaneous tasks where the global configuration of the stimuli is relevant (Mammarela et al., 2008, p. 15). Tests that structure tasks on this organization of the VSWM offer more detailed information on the competencies possessed by children and therefore allow the organization of good methods of intervention. The *BVS-Corsi* battery (Mammarella et al., 2008) is structured in this direction and is organized on two levels of tests. The first level is useful for initial screening of visual-spatial skills, the tests used are the *Corsi Test* and the *Span di Cifre*. Second level tests include active and passive VSWM tests, with sequential and simultaneous tasks. Its structuring allows in-depth evaluation of the components of the VSWM.

FINAL CONSIDERATIONS AND RESEARCH PERSPECTIVES

The relation between Visual-Spatial Working Memory (VSWM) and mental images has been widely accredited by the scientific reference community (Mammarella, 2008). The ability to transform and manipulate mental images sees VSWM also involved in navigational and spatial orientation skills (Garden et al., 2002), in learning semantic knowledge about objects, in decoding visual and spatial coordinates (Hanley et al., 1991) and in non-verbal communication (Doherty-Sneddon, et al., 2001).

For this reason, good performance of VSWM seems to be correlated with good academic results in all those disciplines in which visual-spatial ability are decisive as mathematics, geometry, sciences, drawing, geography (Mammarella et al., 2008). Going into details, the visual-spatial difficulties in nature affect the capacity of alignment and put in columns the mathematical operations, in the reading and writing of a mathematical sign, in the rest and in the carried over of an amount, in the recall and execution of arithmetic procedures (Mammarella et al., 2008).

In the field of geometry, it is possible to observe difficulties in understanding and remembering geometric shapes and in the mental manipulation of forms. For the resolution of geometrics' tasks, it is necessary, in fact, to know how to recall the properties of the geometric figure, and be able to reproduce and operate transformations of it. These are all activities that require processing and manipulation of the mental image of the geometric object (Lucangeli, Mammarella, 2010).

In reference to other scientific disciplines, several are the implications of VSWM in their learning. The skills involved here can call into question the ability to observe reality in a precise and punctual way, to realize space-time changes, to build cause-effect relationships and to integrate graphics and tables (Mammarella et al., 2008, p. 23). The drawing reveals critical issues in the organization of space and topological relationships between the elements.

As a result of poor handling skills of the mental representation of objects, poverty emerges in the graphic execution relative to the representation of details (Mammarella et al., 2008). The same difficulties in spatial relationships between objects are found in the learning of geography where the processing of visual-spatial information is necessary for orientation, for the correct use of topological concepts, for the reproduction of path, etc. (Mammarella et al., 2008).

Furthermore, recent studies highlight the role that VSWM would seem to play in understanding the text. The control and the integration of interferences (literary and implicit), necessary for the construction of meaning during the reading of a text (Giaconi, Capellini, 2015), seems to be charged to the WM, and in particular, of the verbal one, involved in the maintenance and elaboration of verbal and textual stimuli. The VSWM would be activated, instead, in understanding the text when it is accompanied by images (Gyselinck et al., 2002) or when the text describes spatial configurations (Denis, 1996). Recent studies, conducted in this direction, support the hypothesis of a shared system between VSWM and Linguistic Working Memory in the generation of inferences in visual narrative texts, such as the comic strip (Magliano et al., 2016).

The relevance of the visual-spatial abilities in the students' educational success throw down important pedagogical challenges concerning both the rethinking of the teaching of the aforementioned disciplines (Lucangeli, Mammarella 2018; Grimaldi et al., 2012), and the activation of prevention paths (Giaconi, Capellini, 2015) that can be articulated, first, in action to inform, and then in a training for parents and teachers (*Ivi*) about the implications of VSWM in the construction of skills and competences. Therefore, pedagogical emergencies are opening up in the realization of observation tools to detect difficulties and criticalities that are valid, reliable and sustainable such as the study presented in this paper. The activation of a "house to house" screening and the detection of the difficulties in the visual-spatial abilities will be aimed at the design of educational inclusive of strengthening the whole class group paths (*Ibidem,* p. 92) to the benefit not only of students with probable configurations of SpLDs or Nonverbal Learning Disorder but for all. From these considerations, we are going to present a future research path in the Italian context aimed at investigating the correlation between VSMW, reading and writing learning and the related performance. The trial will be conducted with eight years old children attending the second grade of primary school. Students will be subjected to the following tests: *The Rey Complex Figure* test, *Visual-*

Motor Integration test, the *Test of visual perception and visual-motor integration* and *BVS-Corsi* battery.

The research will be conducted during the 2020-2021 school year and it will take place two administrations: at the begging of the school year (September 2020) and after six months (March 2021). The results will allow us to see the role of perceptual and motor performances in the reading and writing learning process and the presence of any critical signals will be used to deepen the comprehensive assessment of Dyslexia and Dysgraphia mixed framework.

REFERENCES

Baddeley, A. D. 1986. *Working Memory*. Oxord: Oxford University Press.

Baddeley, A. D., and Hitch G. J. 1974. "Working memory". In *Recent Advances in Learning and Motivation*, edited by G.A. Bower, 47-90. New York: Academic Press.

Beery, K. E., and Buktenica, N. A. 2000. *VMI, Developmental Test of Visual-Motor Integration*. Florence: Organizzazioni Speciali.

Caffarra, P., Vezzadini, G., Dieci F., Zonato, F., and Venneri A. 2001. "Rey-Osterrieth complex figure: normative values in an Italian population sample". *Neurological Science* 22: 443-447.

Cornoldi, C., and Vecchi, T. 2003. *Visuospatial working memory and individual differences*. Hove: Psychology Press.

Denis, M. 1996. "Imagery and the description of spatial configurations". In *Models of visual-spatial cognition*, edited by M. de Vega, M. J. Intons-Peterson, P. M. Johnson Laird, M. Denis, and M. Marschark, 128-197. London: Oxford University Press.

Doherty-Sneddong, G., Bonner, L., and Bruce V. 2001. "Cognitive demands of face monitoring: evidence for visuospatial overload". *Memory & Cognition* 29: 909-919.

Fastame, M. C., and Antonini, R. 2011. *Recupero in... percorsi e attività per la scuola primaria e secondaria di primo grado*. Trento: Erickson. [*Remediation in...paths and activities for primary and secondary schools*. Trento: Erickson].

Frosting, M., Lefever, D. W., and Whittlesey, J. R. B. 1974. *Developmental of Visual Perception*. Florence: Organizzazioni Speciali.

Garden, S., Cornoldi, C., Logie, R. H. 2002. "Visuo-spatial working memory in navigation". *Applied Cognitive Psychology* 16: 35-50.

Giaconi, C., and Capellini, S. A. 2015. *Conoscere per includere. Riflessioni e linee operative per professionisti in formazione*. [*Know to include. Reflections and operative lines for professionals in training*]. Milano: FrancoAngeli.

Grimaldi, R., Grimaldi, B. S., Marcianò, G., Palmieri, S., Siega, S. 2012. "Robotica educativa e potenziamento delle abilità visuo-spaziali" ["Educational robotics and visual-spatial skills enhancement"]. In *Didamatica 2012*, edited by T. Rosselli, A. Androico, F. Berni, P. Di Bitonto, Rossano V., 1-10. Bari: Aica, Bari.

Gyselinck, V., Dubois-Bouchet, V., Cornoldi, C., De Beni, R., and Ehrlich 2002. "Visuospatial memory and phonological loop in learning from multimedia". *Applied Cognitive Psychology* 16 (VI): 665- 685.

Hammill, D. D., and Pearson, N. A., Voress, J. K. 1994. *TPV, Test di Percezione Visiva e Integrazione Visuo-motoria* [*Visual Perception Test and Visuo-motor Integration*]. Trento: Erickson.

Hanley, J. R., Young, A. W., Pearson, N. A. 1991. "Impairment of the visuospatial sketch pad". *Quarterly Journal of Experimental Psychology* 43: 101-125.

Logie, R. H. 1995. *Visuo-spatial working memory*. Hove: Lawrence Erlbaum Associates.

Lucangeli, D., and Mammarella, I. C. 2010. *Psicologia della cognizione numerica. Approcci teorici, valutazione e intervento* [*Psychology of *numerical cognition. Theoretica approaches, evaluation and intervention*]. Milano: FrancoAngeli.

Magliano, J. P., Larson, A. L., Higgs, K., Loschky, L. C. 2016. "The relative roles of visuospatial and linguistic working memory systems in generating inferences during visual narrative comprehension". *Memory & Cognition* 44 (II): 207-219.

Mammarella, I. C., Toso, C., Pazzaglia, F., and Cornoldi C. 2008. *BVS-Corsi. Batteria per la valutazione della memoria visiva e spaziale.* [*BVS-Corsi. Battery for the evaluation of visual and spatial memory*]. Trento: Erickson.

Mammarella, I. C. 2008. "La Memoria di Lavoro Visuo-Spaziale: una rassegna di studi recenti" ["The Visuo-Spatial Working Memory: a Review of Recent Studies"]. *Giornale italiano di psicologia* 3: 509-540.

Rey, A. 1967. *Reattivo della Figura Complessa* [*Complex Figure Reactive*]. Florence: Organizzazioni Speciali.

Reynolds, C. R., and Bigler, E. D. 1985. *TEMA, Test di Memoria e Apprendimento* [*TEMA, Memory and Learning Test*]. Trento: Erikson.

Siegel, L. S., Ryan, E. B. 1989. "The development of working memory in normally achieving and subtypes of learning disabled children". *Child Development* 60: 973-980.

Thurstone, L. L., and Thurstone T. G. 1985. *PMA, Abilità Mentali Primarie* [*Primary Mental Ability*]. Firenze: Organizzazioni Speciali.

Zaccaria, S. 2008. "Memoria di lavoro attiva e Disturbo da Deficit di Attenzione/Iperattività: una rassegna e una meta-analisi". ["Active Working Memory and Attention Deficit/ Hyperactivity Disorder: a review and a met-analysis"] *Psicologia clinica dello sviluppo* 1: 7-24.

In: Dyslexia
Editors: Catia Giaconi et al.
ISBN: 978-1-53617-593-6
© 2020 Nova Science Publishers, Inc.

Chapter 10

DYSLEXIA IN THE UNIVERSITY SYSTEM: TECHNOLOGY FOR AUTONOMY

Noemi Del Bianco[1], Catia Giaconi[1], Ilaria D'Angelo[1] and Simone Aparecida Capellini[2]
[1]Department of Education, Cultural Heritage and Tourism,
University of Macerata (UNIMC), Macerata, Italy
[2]Investigation Learning Disabilities Laboratory (LIDA),
Department of Speech and Hearing Sciences,
São Paulo State University
"Júlio de Mesquita Filho" (UNESP),
Marilia, São Paulo, Brazil

INTRODUCTION

Specific Learning Disorders (SpLDs) are identified as organic-based neurological disorders with an evolutionary trend and the most common types "are those that impact the areas of reading, math, and written expression" (Cortiella & Horowitz, 2014, p. 3), with the appearance of slowing down and/or an atypia in comparison to the normal trend (Dehaene, 2009; Gérard, 2011). SpLDs, that include Dyslexia, are described as "unexpected, significant difficulties in academic achievement and related areas of learning" (Cortiella & Horowitz, 2014, p. 3). We agree with Zappaterra (2016) that "such issues become even more urgent in the university context" (Zappaterra, 2016, p. 122).

In this direction, various studies and practices (Capellini et al., 2018; de Anna & Covelli, 2018; Giaconi et al., 2018) have focused on the potential of Information and Communication Technologies, to enable, extend and also enhance students learning within the college field. In general, digital technologies can become an integral aspect of the University student experience, since they are useful in the process of "supporting students' organization of academic work and general ability to 'manage academic demands'" (Henderson et al., 2017, p. 1576). As stated in other works (Giaconi et al., 2018), "the technological sector has a great potential to explore and improve accessibility" (Giaconi et al., 2018, p. 196) concerning both materials and contents, allowing also students with Dyslexia to achieve positive results in college.

Research shows that the use of technologies in educational/training processes allows an increase in motivation to study and the personalization of learning (Pavone, 2010), in addition to favoring the development of greater personal independence and inclusive participation (Henderson et al., 2017; Giaconi et al., 2018).

Studies (Griffith, 2008; Park et al., 2014) have demonstrated the importance of motivation for learning, where "the incorporation of technologies, such as the use of computers in the learning process, represents a highly motivational factor for the development of academic abilities" (Capellini et al., 2018, p. 74). Because hardware and software instruments integrate texts, images, audio and videos, students can use technological resources interactively, benefiting from a series of stimuli, keeping them involved during their learning time. In addition, technologies are part of the students' daily life, and for this reason can become an excellent resource to increase their motivation (Capellini et al., 2018).

The interactive nature of technological devices, with input suited to the person's needs, represents another turning point to achieve the learning process. The flexibility that characterizes technologies allow the correct identification of the most appropriate tool for personal characteristics, "in accordance with the tasks to be performed, the context and the degree of acceptability tolerated by the user" (Giaconi et al., 2018, p. 198). Personalized, adaptive and suitable tools can allow the activation of educational processes, affecting the styles and rhythms of learning of each student (Besio, 2005, p. 142); the plurality of communication channels can make possible to act, manage and shape materials and contents in relation to one's personal needs. Technologies, allowing differentiated educational performances for students who present SpLDs, implement relational and emotional approaches to knowledge, encouraging metacognitive processes that allow them to increase their knowledge levels.

Among the positive aspects that can be highlighted, in connection with the use of technological devices by students with SpLDs at the University, there is also the potential of support that allows the implementation of independent and autonomous learning. The possibility that technology offers to develop a more active role within the University context increases student's involvement in learning and, consequently, develops their autonomy (Giaconi et al., 2018). Technological tools can help all students at all levels of education "to complete their work more easily and independently" (Giaconi et al., 2018, p. 76).

TECHNOLOGIES AND ACADEMIC TRAINING

The use of technologies in the higher education system allows also the promotion of equity in learning and training opportunities (Henderson et al., 2017; Giaconi et al., 2018), that represents the keystone of an inclusive educational process. ICTs, entering in the academic contexts are able to favor the activation of inclusive dynamics, expanding social contexts, with the goal of promoting the full participation of all students while respecting different needs and abilities.

In Italian experiences, there are to academics training for students with SpLDs, and specifically with Dyslexia, in the University (Giaconi & Capellini, 2015; Giaconi et al., 2018).

We also agree with the reference literature (Cornoldi et al., 2010; Friso et al., 2011; Giaconi & Capellini, 2015; Cajola & Traversetti, 2017) that the management and planning of the study method represent the first compensatory tool par excellence for students with SpLDs. In this direction, the technologies to be used for study support can be plural, in order to guarantee both organizational aids and visual supports.

An example of an App that "plan the habitus for the study", increasing how to manage and create a complete step-by-step study system could be CanDue (iOS, Android). Among the useful devices for studying can be identified tools and Apps for "NoteTaking" "Audio Recording" and "Audio Transcription Services & Apps." Instead, to increase visual organization and thinking, improving comprehension and retention with images, there are several Apps that help in the creation of "Maps." Even the possibility to transform text from handwriting to a digital format could be realized thanks to different technological tools.

Focusing specifically on the issues related to SpLDs, as stated by the "National Center for Learning Disabilities (NCLD)" in "The State of Learning Disabilities" (Cortiella & Horowitz, 2014), the areas of reading, written and math expression are identified as the most critical. For these reasons, in the academic path of these students, some technological tools can be of fundamental help in order to compensate for their Disorders.

In terms of reading expression, considering that students express difficulties with «phonemic awareness (the ability to notice, think about and work with individual sounds in words); phonological processing (detecting and discriminating differences in phonemes or speech sounds); difficulties with word decoding, fluency, rate of reading, rhyming, spelling, vocabulary, comprehension and written expression» (Cortiella & Horowitz, 2014, p. 3).

There are Apps that can be identified as useful for them because they can transform "Text into Speech." For students with Disorders in writing, it can be hard to capture both the physical act of writing and the quality of written expression. Common characteristics include: «tight, awkward pencil grip and body position; tiring quickly while writing, and avoiding writing or drawing tasks; trouble forming letter shapes as well as inconsistent spacing between letters or words; difficulty writing or drawing on a line or within margins; trouble organizing thoughts on paper; trouble keeping track of thoughts already written down; difficulty with syntax structure and grammar; large gap between written ideas and understanding demonstrated through speech» (Cortiella & Horowitz, 2014, p. 4). In this direction, in the technological market, there are many Apps that convert "Speech to Text" for students that are struggling with written expression.

For further details, we summarize in the table below "Table 1" examples of some tools/Apps that can be used by all students, also with SpLDs, to support them during their academic career.

Table 1. Examples of tools/Apps useful for University students with SpLDs

Areas to be supported	Examples of tools/Apps
Management and Organization	"Time Management Organizers" Apps: Chipper by Cram (iOS, Android); My Students Life (iOS, Android); Study Planner (iOS, Android); StudySmart-Study organizer (iOS, Android). "Task" Apps: Apple Reminders (iOS); Clear (iOS, Android); Google Tasks (online, iOS, Android); Pocket Lists (iOS, Android). "Memos" Apps: Apple Notes (iOS); Google Keep (online, iOS, Android); Simplenote (online, iOS, Android).
Method of Study	"Habitus for the study" Apps: CanDue (iOS, Android); iHomework (iOS); istudiezpro (iOS); MyHomework (online, iOS, Android); Shovel (iOS, Android). "NoteTaking" and "Audio Recording" tools: MS OneNote; Notability; Otter AI; Smart Pens; TranscribeMe! "Maps" Apps Cmap (online, Android); Connected Mind (online); DropMind (online, iOS); Inspiration (software iOS, Windows, App iOS); iThoughts HD (iOS); MindNode (iOS); Mindly (online, Android); SimpleMind (online, iOS, Android).

Areas to be supported	Examples of tools/Apps
	"Handwriting to digital format" tools:
	Aegir SmartPen with Livescribe+ (Android);
	Galaxy Note 8 & higher (Android);
	Notability w/iPad (iOS);
	Pen to Print, (iOS, Android).
Reading	"Text to Speech" Apps:
	Beeline Reader (online);
	Google Read Aloud (online, iOS, Android);
	Kurzweil (iOS, Android);
	Mac Reader (iOS);
	MS Immersive Reader (iOS, Android);
	Natural Reader (online, iOS, Android);
	Read & Write Gold (iOS, Android);
	RWG extensions for FF & Chrome (online);
	Windows Text to Speech (online, iOS, Android).
Writing	"Speech to Text" Apps:
	Co: Writer (online, iOS, Android);
	Draft: builder (online, iOS, Android).
	Dragon Naturally Speaking (Android);
	Mac Dictate (iOS);
	Otter AI (iOS, Android);
	Windows Speech Recognition (iOS, Android).
	"Editing and Research" Apps:
	Grammarly (online, iOS, Android);
	LiquidText (iOS);
	Read Write Gold (online, iOS, Android);
	Zotero (online, iOS, Android).

CONCLUSION

The use of technological supports by University students with SpLDs leads our reflection to make a pedagogical analysis. Despite the positive aspects that emerged in the previous sections, some critiques need to be underlined.

Considering that the availability of these tools, or their simple operational use, alone do not guarantee practices of effective learning or educational success in the academic field, technological tools and Apps that have been presented in this paper represent a compensatory support for the students, to be used in some cases and/or for specific contexts. As stated by Henderson et al., (2017) the use of digital technologies for learning varies between subject disciplines, levels of study, modes of delivery and institutions. For this reason, it is difficult to see a complete survey of all the technologies present in the digital market, in close correlation with the contents of the courses and above all in reference to the peculiarities linked to the specific and personal nuances of the SpLDs and Dyslexia. The technological world is proceeding with extreme speed in the creation of new proposals, which, if these products are properly designed, they can be modified and never definitive. Therefore, in this paper, a complete and exhaustive review of all the existing devices in the technological field has not been determined, but rather examples have been proposed in relation to the support modalities of some learning difficulties during the University course.

Considering the vastness and the constantly evolving technological proposals, knowing which devices are present in the market, recognizing the tools that are the most useful related to issues of clarity and flexibility in achieving one's 'learning' goals (Virtanen & Lindblom-Ylänne, 2010), can be difficult in practice. Students could, in fact, find themselves lacking in information and forms of counseling that allows them to fully grasp the potential and/or negativity of instruments in relation to their personal peculiarities. For these reasons, the need for a guide emerges, which is a pedagogical support, able to answer to issues of functionality, responsiveness and ease of being able to find one's way around the demands (Douglas et al., 2015). The work methodologies supported by the ICTs show how they do not replace nor complete 'exhaustively' the work that the student has to carry out since on their own and without pedagogical support technologies do not represent the solution to the difficulties that students encounter (de Anna & Covelli, 2018). Specifically, it is necessary that educational practices are aimed to, on the one hand, guarantee the technical use of technology, or the possibility of resorting to experts when necessary, on the other, increase the autonomous preparation of the student, both in the search for devices, and use of the instruments. These pedagogical training proposals, calibrated both in relation to the specific needs of each student and to the academic requests, concern University services, teaching staff and national policies, since they are able to activate educational methods that can be supportive in this direction.

A further weak point that we want to highlight is connected to the sustainability of the expenditure and the costs of some devices. In some cases, the use of technologically advanced and particularly excellent software and Apps require payment and the costs are not always moderate. In this direction, the technology does not seem to be accessible to many students, who prefer to avoid the use of some tools, rather than pay for their use. Even in these cases, we would like to urge greater sensitivity to this issue to University services, but above all to national policies, which in a much more advantageous way, can purchase licenses and equipment for the whole student body.

The high number of students with disabilities and SpLDs attending Universities, and the exponential growth of the technological proposals present in the digital market, push our reflection to underline the need for further research calibrated to the possibilities that technology can offer in relation to the realization of a system adaptable for each student. In this direction, as expressed in other works (Giaconi et al., 2018), it is necessary to create an integrated system of devices to be used in University contexts. An aggregate system of useful Apps or tools would, in fact, facilitate access and organization, with the aim of allowing even students with Dyslexia to have a more fluid and direct use of resources.

Finally, the substantial area of development and implementation of technological products drives us to reflect on the missing data concerning students' personal perceptions in relation to their use of technology in the academic world for learning purposes. Future research could explore the effects of technology in learning principles, to understand better the use of technology in higher education thanks to rigorous empirical studies. Knowing the students' perspective would also enable them to test materials and improve their skills.

REFERENCES

Besio, S. 2005. *Tecnologie assistive per la disabilità. [Assistive technologies for disability]*. Lecce: Pensa MultiMedia.

Burgstahler, S. 2015. *Universal Design in Higher Education: From Principles to Practice*. 2nd edition. Harvard: Harvard University Press.

Cajola, L.C., and Traversetti, M. 2017. "Il metodo di studio come prima misura compensativa per l'inclusione degli allievi con DSA; progetto di ricerca." ["The study method as the first compensatory measure for the inclusion of students with DSA; research project."] *Journal of Educational cultural and Psychological Studies* 14: 127-151.

Capellini, S. A., Franco dos Santos Liporaci, G., Sellin, L., Herrera Cardoso, M., Giaconi, C., and Del Bianco, N. 2018. "Inclusion and New Technology for Students with Learning Disorders and Attention Deficit with Hyperactivity Disorder." *Education Sciences & Society* 9(1): 73-80.

Cortiella, C. and Horowitz, S. H. 2014. *The State of Learning Disabilities: Facts, Trends and Emerging Issues*. New York: National Center for Learning Disabilities.

Cornoldi, C., De Beni, R., and Gruppo MT. 2001. *Imparare a studiare* 2 [*Learn to study* 2]. Trento: Erickson.

Douglas, J., Douglas, A., McClelland, R., and Davies, J. 2015. "Understanding Student Satisfaction and Dissatisfaction: An Interpretive Study in the UK Higher Education Context." *Studies in Higher Education* 40(2): 329-349.

Dehaene, S. 2009. *I neuroni della lettura* [*The neurons of reading*]. Milano: Raffaello Cortina.

de Anna, L., and Covelli, A. 2018. "La Didattica inclusiva nell'Università: innovazione e successo formativo degli studenti con Special Educational Needs." ["Inclusive Didactics in the University: innovation and educational success of students with Special Educational Needs."] *Form@re - Open Journal per la formazione in rete* 18(1): 333-345.

Friso G., Amadio V., Paiano A., Russo M.R., and Cornoldo C. 2011. *Studio Efficace per ragazzi con DSA* [*Effective Study for Kids with Specific Learning Disorders*]. Trento: Erickson.

Giaconi, C., and Capellini, S. A. 2015. *Conoscere per includere* [*Know to include*]. FrancoAngeli: Milano.

Giaconi, C., Capellini, S. A., Del Bianco, N., Taddei, A., and D'Angelo, I. 2018. "Study Empowerment for inclusion." *Education Sciences & Society* 9(2):166-183.

Giaconi, C., and Del Bianco, N. 2018. "Didattica universitaria e dispositivi tecnologici inclusivi: il progetto Inclusione 3.0." In *In Azione: prove di Inclusione* ["University teaching and inclusive technological devices: The Inclusion 3.0 project."], edited by C., Giaconi, N., Del Bianco, 284-295. Milan: FrancoAngeli.

Gérard, C.-L. 2011. *Cliniques des troubles des apprentissages. De l'évaluation neuropsychologique à la programmation educative* [*Learning Disorders Clinics. From neuropsychological assessment to educational programming*]. Bruxelles: De Boeck. Education.

Griffiths, C. 2008. *Lessons from good language learners*. Cambridge: Cambridge University Press.

Heiman, T., and Precel, K. 2003. "Students with learning disabilities in higher education." *Journal of Learning Disabilities* 36: 248-260.

Henderson, M., Selwyn, N., and Aston, R. 2017. "What works and why? Student perceptions of 'useful' digital technology in university teaching and learning." *Studies in Higher Education* 42(8): 1567-1579.

Kirkland, J. 2009. "The development of protocols for assessment and intervention at university for students with dyslexia." In *The Routledge companion to dyslexia*, edited by G. Reid, 261-264. New York: Routledge/Taylor & Francis Group.

Meyer, A., and O'Neil, L. 2000. "Beyond access: Universal design for learning." *The Exceptional Parent* 30(3): 59-61.

Moriarty, M. A. 2007. "Inclusive Pedagogy: Teaching Methodologies to Reach Diverse Learners in Science Instruction." *Equity & Excellence in Education* 40: 252-265.

Pavone, M. 2010. *Dall'esclusione all'inclusione* [*From exclusion to inclusion*]. Milano: Mondadori.

Pavone, M., and Bellacicco R. 2016. "University: a universe of study and independent living opportunities for students with disabilities. Goals and critical issues." *Education Sciences & Research* 7(1): 101-120.

Park, B., Plass, J., and Brünken, R. 2014. "Cognitive and affective processes in multimedia learning." *Learning and Instruction* 29: 125-127.

Pino, M., and Mortari, L. 2014. "The Inclusion of Students with Dyslexia in Higher Education: A Systematic Review Using Narrative Synthesis." *Dyslexia* 20: 346-369.

Rivera C. J., Wood C. L, James M., and Williams S. 2019. "Improving Study Outcomes for College Students with Executive Functioning Challenges." *Career Development and Transition for Exceptional Individuals* 42(3): 139-147.

Rose, D. H., and Meyer, A. 2002. "Teaching every student in the digital age: Universal design for learning." *Association for Supervision and Curriculum Development*. Alexandria, VA

Sala, I., Sánchez Fuentes, I., Giné. C., and Díez Villoria, E. 2014. "Análisis de los distintos enfoques del paradigma del diseño universal aplicado a la educación." ["Analysis of the different approaches of the paradigm of universal design applied to education."] *Revista Latinoamericana de Inclusión Educativa* 8(1): 143-152.

Silver, P., Bourke, A., and Strehorn, K. C. 1998. "Universal instructional design in higher education: an approach for inclusion." *Equity & Excellence in Education* 31(2): 47-51.

Stacey, G., and Singleton, C. 2003. "Dyslexia support in higher education in the United Kingdom." In *Learning disabilities in higher education and beyond*, edited by S. A., Vogel, G., Vogel, V., Sharoni, and O. Dahan, 45-68. Baltimore: York Press.

Virtanen, V., and Lindblom-Ylänne, S. 2010. "University Students' and Teachers' Conceptions of Teaching and Learning in the Biosciences." *Instructional Science* 38(4): 355-70.

Zappaterra, T. 2016. "Dyslexia in the University. Guidelines for inclusion and teaching of the University of Florence." *Education Sciences & Society* 7(1): 121-137.

Web References

Australian Government Department of Education & Training, (2016), 2015 Appendix 2 – Equity groups; from https://docs.education.gov.au/documents/2015-appendix-2-equity-groups [October, 10, 2019].

Censis, (2017), Processi formativi, 51° Rapporto sulla situazione sociale del Paese/201 (Report 2017) [Censis, (2017), Training processes, 51st Report on the country's social situation/201 (Report 2017)]; from http://www.censis.it/ rapporto-annuale/ 51%C2%B0-rapporto-sulla-situazione-sociale-del-paese2017 [October, 10, 2019].

Convention on the Rights of Persons with Disabilities, https://www.unric.org/html/italian/pdf/Convenzione-disabili-ONU.pdf [October, 10, 2019].

Higher Education Statistics Agency [HESA]. (nd). UK domiciled student enrollments by disability and sex, Academic years 2014/15

to 2017/18. Retrieved from https://www.hesa.ac.uk/data-and-analysis/students/whos-in-he/characteristics [October, 10, 2019].
https://europa.eu/rapid/press-release_MEMO-10-200_it.htm [October, 10, 2019].
https://softwarelicense.arizona.edu/students [October, 10, 2019].
http://udloncampus.cast.org/ [October, 10, 2019].
https://www.azed.gov/specialeducation/at/ [October, 10, 2019].
https://www.w3.org/WAI/test-evaluate/tools/selecting/#top [October, 10, 2019].
U.S. Department of Education, National Center for Education Statistics, (2019), *Digest of Education Statistics, 2017* (NCES 2018-070), Table 311.10; from https://nces.ed.gov/fastfacts/display.asp?id=60 [October, 10, 2019].

EDITORS' CONTACT INFORMATION

Catia Giaconi
Full Professor of Didactics and Special Pedagogy
Department of Education, Cultural Heritage and Tourism
at the University of Macerata
Email: catia.giaconi@unimc.it

Simone Aparecida Capellini
Investigation Learning Disabilities Laboratory (LIDA),
Full-Professor at Department of Speech and Hearing Sciences,
São Paulo State University "Júlio de Mesquita Filho" (UNESP),
Marília, São Paulo, Brazil
Email: sacap@uol.com.br

INDEX

A

academic difficulties, 38
academic performance, 85, 86, 89, 90, 91, 92, 93, 97, 98, 101
alphabetic principle, 23, 30, 31, 35, 36
American Psychiatric Association (APA), 2, 10, 93, 98, 104
articulation, 19, 112
assessment, 1, 23, 25, 26, 33, 37, 38, 40, 45, 72, 84, 94, 98, 106, 110, 115, 129, 130
assessment procedures, 84
assessment tools, 110
assistive technology, 3, 8, 9
Attention Deficit Hyperactivity Disorder, 92
auditory element (phoneme), 7, 16, 17, 18, 19, 20, 30, 34, 35, 36, 38, 39, 44, 55, 56

B

behavioral problems, 2
behaviors, 84

C

children, 2, 6, 7, 11, 12, 22, 23, 27, 38, 39, 40, 56, 68, 80, 87, 88, 93, 94, 105, 106, 107, 113, 115, 118
Chinese Language, vi, ix, 71, 72, 73, 76, 79
coordination, 84, 86, 87, 88, 89, 91, 92, 94, 97, 102, 103, 106, 109

D

decoding, 2, 5, 8, 16, 23, 24, 27, 30, 36, 43, 44, 60, 61, 62, 84, 113, 123
deficiency(ies), 2, 17, 106
deficit, 16, 33, 56, 59, 65, 66, 67, 84, 86, 94, 96, 103, 105, 106
Department of Education, 109, 131, 132, 133
developmental dyslexia, vi, x, 18, 39, 45, 55, 56, 59, 61, 62, 64, 65, 66, 81, 84, 85, 86, 94, 95
diagnostic criteria, 56
differential diagnosis, 85
digital technologies, 120, 126

disability, 128, 131
discrimination, 38, 43, 55, 109
discrimination training, 38
disorder, 1, 2, 16, 56, 60, 67, 86, 94, 105, 106
dysgraphia, 84, 89, 90, 91, 92, 93, 115
dyslexia, v, vi, vii, ix, x, 1, 2, 3, 8, 9, 11, 12, 13, 15, 18, 19, 22, 30, 32, 36, 37, 38, 39, 40, 41, 43, 45, 47, 48, 49, 50, 51, 52, 53, 54, 55, 56, 57, 59, 60, 61, 63, 64, 65, 66, 67, 68, 69, 71, 72, 73, 74, 75, 76, 77, 79, 80, 81, 82, 83, 84, 85, 86, 89, 90, 91, 92, 93, 94, 95, 96, 97, 98, 100, 101, 102, 103, 104, 105, 106, 107, 115, 119, 120, 122, 126, 127, 130, 131

E

educational opportunities, 30, 72
educational practices, 126
educational process, 121, 122
educational psychology, 68
educational research, 67
elementary school, 25, 27, 32, 40, 45, 69, 85
English Language, 26

F

fine motor function, vi, x, 96, 97, 104
fine motor integration, 97, 98, 99, 100, 101, 103
five-syllable non-polysyllabic word repetition, 22
four-syllable non-polysyllabic word repetition, 22

G

genetic background, 103
grapheme-phoneme relationship, 16

H

handwriting, vi, ix, 6, 8, 10, 83, 85, 92, 93, 94, 95, 97, 102, 104, 106, 122, 125
higher education, 122, 127, 129, 131
hyperactivity, 56, 67, 94, 105

I

identification, 18, 19, 20, 24, 30, 34, 36, 37, 44, 45, 54, 55, 60, 68, 121
independent living, 130
individual differences, 28, 116
Information and Communication Technologies (ICTs), 120, 122, 126
intervention, 10, 12, 18, 19, 21, 23, 25, 27, 30, 33, 34, 35, 36, 37, 38, 39, 40, 41, 47, 61, 63, 65, 66, 68, 69, 84, 86, 87, 93, 113, 117, 130
intervention response, 30, 35, 36

K

kindergarten children, 28, 105

L

learning, 1, 2, 3, 6, 9, 10, 11, 12, 16, 17, 23, 27, 28, 30, 37, 40, 56, 57, 61, 62, 65, 66, 67, 68, 69, 72, 73, 76, 79, 80, 84, 96, 97, 103, 106, 109, 110, 113, 114, 115, 117, 118, 120, 121, 122, 125, 126, 127, 129, 130
learning difficulties, 12, 27, 40, 62, 66, 126
learning disabilities, 1, 10, 11, 40, 57, 67, 69, 106, 129
learning process, 2, 96, 97, 103, 115, 120, 121
lexical decision, 46, 47, 49
lexical processing, 65

lexical routes, 46
linguistic processing, 44, 60
literacy, 2, 7, 8, 11, 15, 23, 28, 30, 36, 38, 39, 41, 43, 56, 59, 60, 83, 84
long-term memory, 96

M

Metalinguistic and Reading Skills Protocol, 18
Metalinguistic Skills Protocol – PROHMELE, 19, 20, 21, 22, 25
metaphonological skills, v, ix, 17, 18, 22, 23, 26, 29, 30, 31, 35, 36
motor skills, 84, 91, 92, 93, 94, 95, 97, 98, 102, 103, 104, 107, 111

N

naming, 34, 55, 56, 60, 62, 65, 66, 67, 69
National Center for Education Statistics (NCES), 132
non-trisyllabic word repetition, 22

O

occipital regions, 84

P

parents, 9, 62, 86, 115
phonemes, 7, 8, 16, 17, 29, 30, 80, 123
phonemic segment, 16, 18, 32
phonological awareness, 6, 17, 18, 23, 28, 29, 38, 40, 41, 43, 56, 66, 67
phonological deficit, 8
phonological form, 7
Phonological Intervention Program, 22
prevention, 30, 40, 115
primary school, 40, 115

pronunciation, 44, 74, 79
pseudo word reading, 22
psychology, 28, 37, 38, 41, 94
psychotherapy, 39, 68

Q

quality of life, 3

R

reading, x, 2, 3, 4, 5, 9, 11, 12, 13, 16, 17, 18, 19, 21, 22, 23, 24, 25, 26, 27, 28, 30, 34, 35, 36, 37, 39, 40, 41, 43, 44, 45, 46, 49, 50, 51, 52, 55, 56, 59, 60, 61, 62, 63, 64, 65, 66, 67, 68, 69, 73, 74, 75, 76, 77, 80, 83, 84, 93, 94, 98, 102, 109, 113, 114, 115, 119, 123, 129
reading comprehension, 2, 4, 11, 24, 27, 36, 60, 61, 62, 63, 64, 65, 66, 67, 69
reading comprehension test, 69
reading difficulties, 11, 17, 41, 60
reading disability, 41
reading disorder, 40
reading skills, 18, 25, 68
real and pseudo word reading, 22

S

school learning, 61, 97, 109
specific learning disorders, 119, 129
speech, 5, 8, 16, 17, 23, 33, 40, 45, 56, 66, 86, 123
spelling, 2, 4, 5, 8, 10, 16, 36, 39, 43, 59, 65, 67, 83, 123
syllable addition, 20, 22
syllable substitution, 22

T

task planning, 8
teachers, 9, 26, 60, 75, 79, 86, 115
teaching strategies, 79, 80
technology (ies), 2, 3, 4, 5, 6, 7, 8, 9, 10, 11, 12, 120, 121, 122, 126, 127, 128, 129
training, 6, 28, 38, 41, 57, 71, 115, 117, 120, 122, 127

U

university student, 79, 131

V

visual element (grapheme), 7, 16, 17, 30, 35, 38, 39, 44, 55, 56
visual processing, 44, 60
visual stimuli, 24, 31, 110
visual-space working memory, 110
vocabulary, 2, 4, 44, 69, 123

W

word recognition, 2, 17, 18, 44, 46, 65
word repetition, 22
working memory, 23, 24, 34, 96, 103, 116, 117, 118